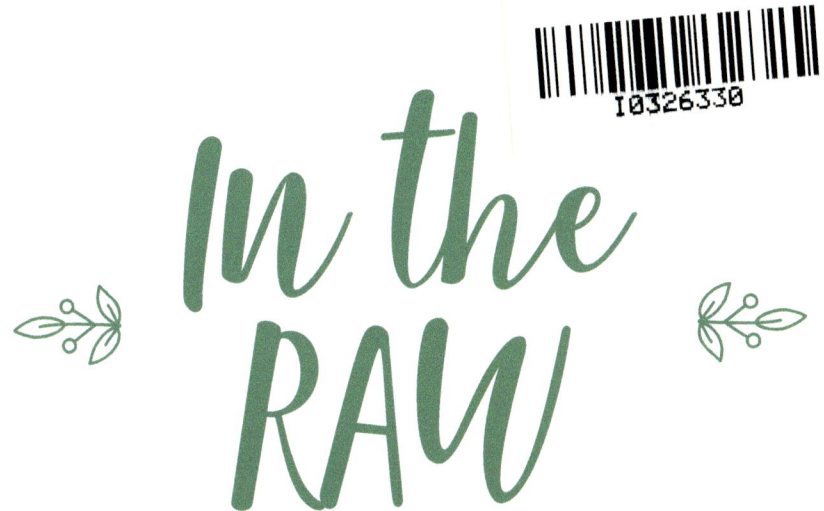

The Healthy Raw Food Manual

Revised 2018 Edition

Anne Clark

Disclaimer

The contents of this book are for information only. This book is not intended to be a substitute for obtaining proper medical advice from a health care professional. Always consult your General Practitioner before making any changes to your nutritional routine. The author, publisher and copyright holder assume no responsibility for any injury, or damage caused or sustained while using nutritional remedies.

Copyright © Anne Clark, 2018

All rights reserved. No part of this publication may be reproduced, stored in a retrieval system, or transmitted in any form by any means, electronic, mechanical, photocopied, recording or otherwise, without prior written permission of the author.

First published 1993.

Reprinted with revisions 1999, 2008, 2010, 2018.

PUBLISHED BY Anne Clark

ISBN: 978-0-9804941-8-1

Photography and art: Anne Clark & Darryl Clark

Edit and design: www.authorsupportservices.com

Printed in Australia

www.anneclark.com.au

This book is dedicated to Darryl and my precious son, Jay.

Thank you to all my loyal customers who encourage me to explore healthy recipes and continue to write these books.

When food is cooked, it will sustain,
but not without its share of pain.
You can look at sprouts with love or hate,
but live food will regenerate.

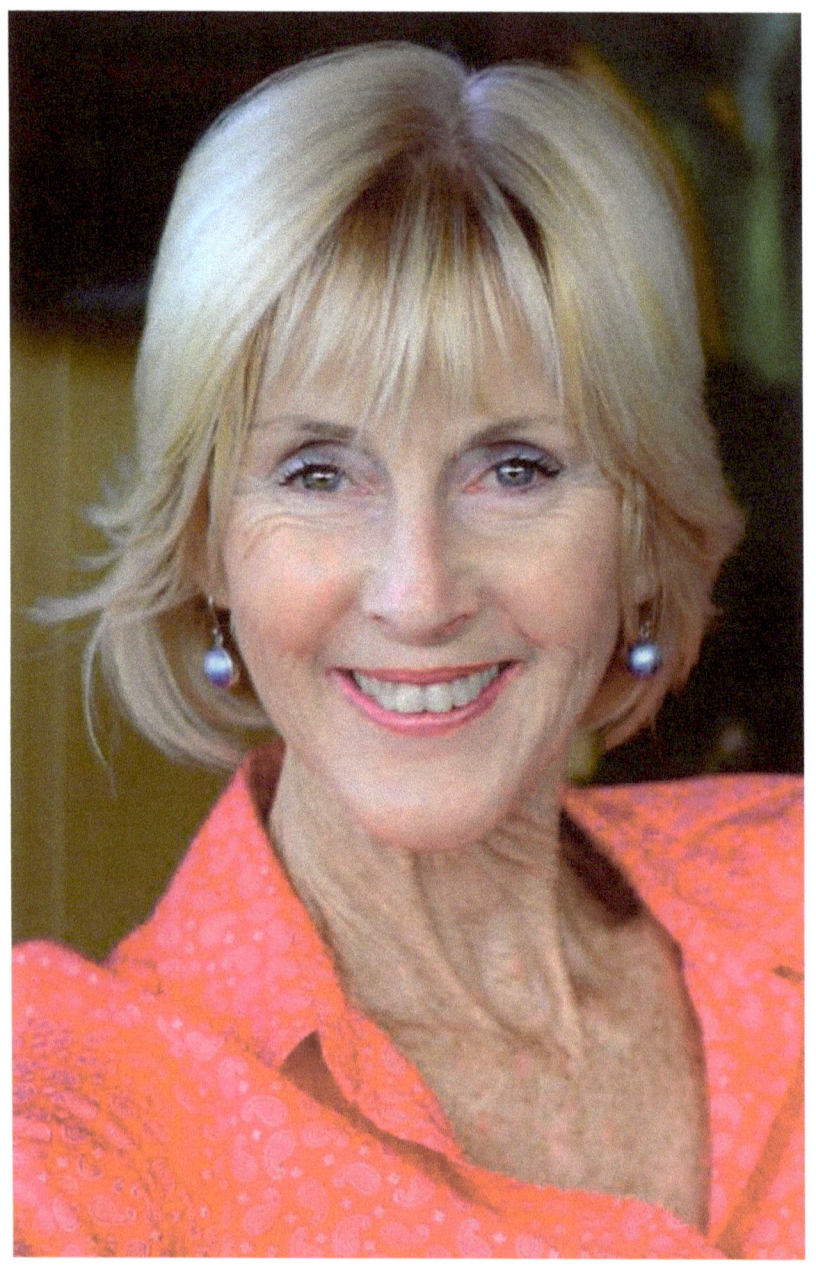

Anne Clark is a lifestyle health consultant, author and speaker. She has been speaking for over 30 years on health and wellbeing and is passionate about sharing her knowledge and empowering others to improve their health and happiness. She has written over 18 books and is a pioneer in healthy eating, being Australia's first raw food author.

With decades of clinical experience, Anne carries out iridology and health evaluations using the Nutri-Energetic System (NES), which treat the distortions and blockages in the body's energy field. She is also one of the original wellness advocates for doTERRA essential oils and enjoys using oils in food and to enhance emotional wellbeing.

Anne regularly runs interactive seminars and workshops on raw food preparation, bowel health, weight management, gut-brain connection, fermented foods and other natural health and lifestyle topics. She is also a speaker on radio and television and guest presents for business networking events around Australia.

Anne believes success in health and life is nothing more than a decision away and that the secret to health and wellbeing is being joyful, achieved by finding something you love to do, loving someone and being loved in return. It is Anne's wish that you find a peaceful place to live within yourself and that you enjoy this book and it helps you to create beautiful food for yourself and the ones you love.

Contact Anne for consultations, workshops and book sales at

www.anneclark.com.au.

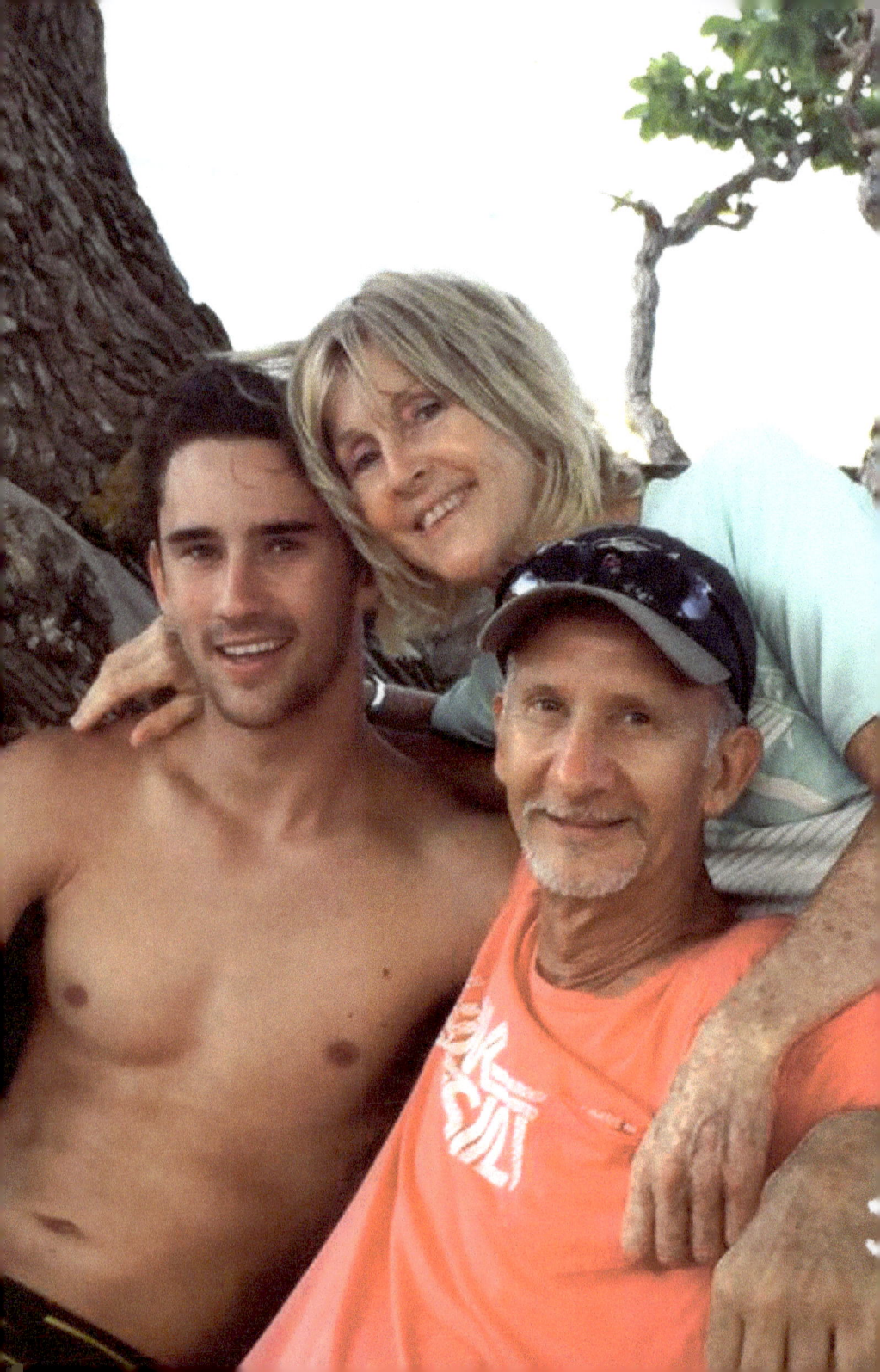

 # Contents

Introduction 1
The philosophy of uncooked food 5
To cook or not to cook 15
A way of eating 19
Detoxification & the three-day clean up 23
Vitamins and minerals 35
Digestion – what's it all about 69
Recipes for Life 85
Cooking tips 211
Ingredients in detail 215
Walking 225
Breathing 231
Posture and alignment 235
Teeth 239
Fasting... gain control of an out-of-control life! 241
Sunbathing 245
Skin brushing 247
Sprouting 249
Living health – ten daily health acts 253
Recipe Index 257
Other books by Anne Clark 261

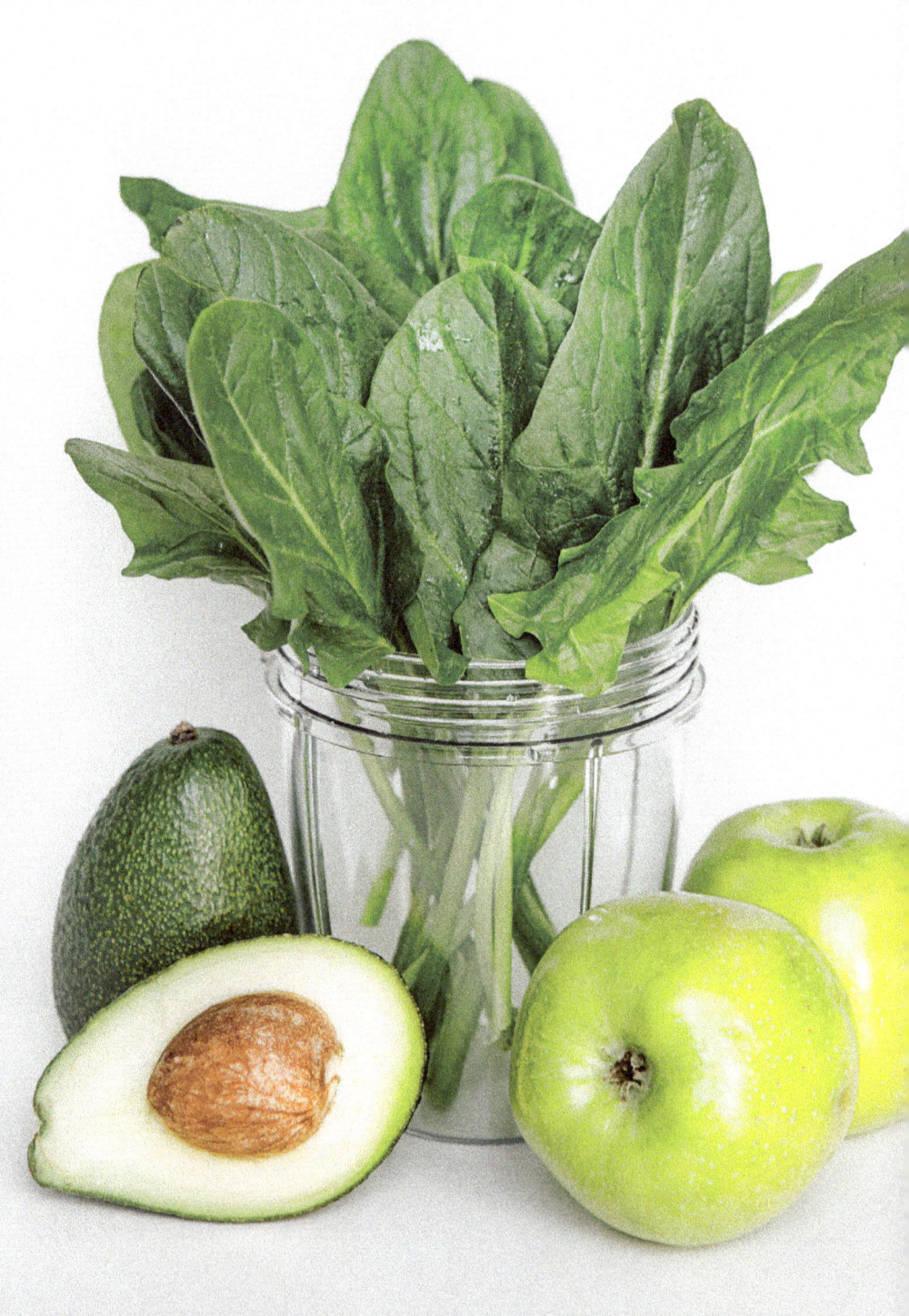

 # Introduction

Hello and welcome to *In the Raw* 2018 edition.

I started taking responsibility for my health many years ago. Gradually, through reading and experimenting with food and food combinations, I excluded all animal products from my diet and discovered the joy of consuming living foods. To me raw food is logical. I think it is ironic that people need to learn about raw foods, how to prepare them and how to cleanse the body, as it really should be second nature. Sadly, it's not second nature to a lot of people and that is why this book is so valuable. Advising people how to eat and prepare healthy raw meals is the easy part, but where the challenge begins is in accepting that there needs to be a change and approaching that change with a positive frame of mind and a willingness to give it a go. When the student is ready, the teacher will come!

Technology has taken us to great limits by enabling us to fly from one part of the world to another. We can flick a switch for power and increase our productivity by using computers. Technology has also contributed to the devastation of our health with the invention of microwave ovens which kill valuable enzymes in our food, refrigerators that keep our food beyond their natural lifetime, and electric lights and televisions which prevent us from going to sleep when the sun goes down and keep us indoors consuming stale air. Eating live, fresh organic food, recycling our waste and going back to basics is where we should be heading. I'm still idealistic enough to believe that where there is hope there is knowledge. We all need to open our minds to a simpler way of living and live food is part of this.

This book will help you to understand more about raw food, fasting, sprouting, walking, body maintenance and self-control. You will learn that raw food is an essential part of a healthy diet and the benefits are enormous! Raw food can help to keep your weight down, increase your vitality and wellbeing, and build your resistance to disease and fatigue. A raw food diet is naturally high in fibre, which makes you feel full and prevents overeating. Your body is also cleansed of stored wastes and toxins, and this aids in the functioning of the digestive system. You will enjoy many of the benefits of raw food by initially using the recipes in this book as part of your regular diet. It is worth changing the balance of cooked to raw until you are eating more raw food than cooked. I still enjoy a freshly baked muffin or slice of bread, but I make sure that I have plenty of fresh high-water-content foods to balance each meal.

I have included a delicious collection of new recipes suitable for children and the whole family. You will also note that there are new recipes in which I have used essential oils. These are certified, pure, therapeutic and food grade oils and useful both in cooking and for enhancing your environment.

Now is the best time to start if you aspire to live a healthy lifestyle. Decide today that you will increase the water content in your food by choosing to eat more live food. Decide today that you will treat your body with the respect it deserves and the rewards will come to you in nature's slow but sure way. *Most importantly, have fun with the concept of raw food and live to enjoy your life.*

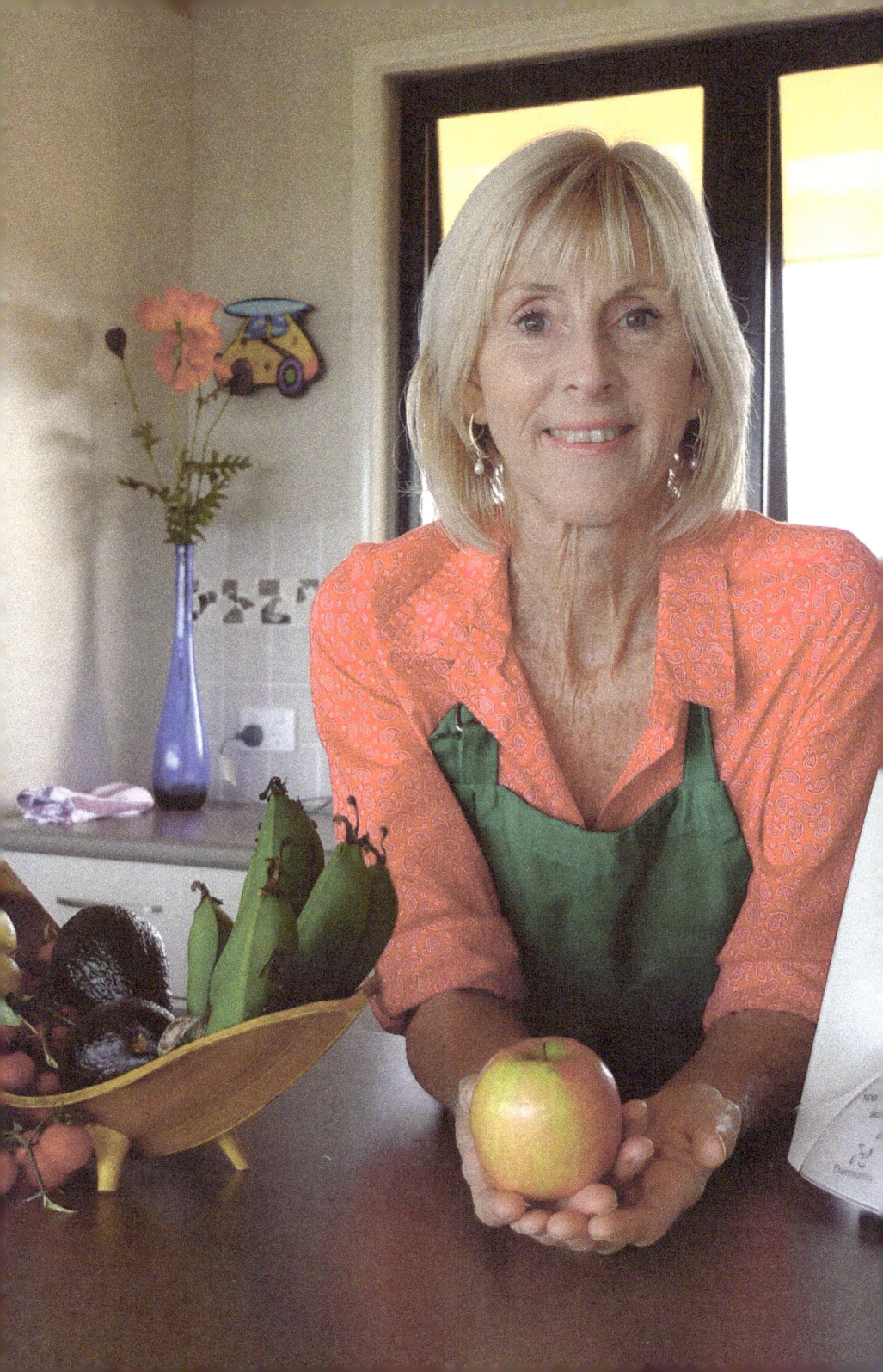

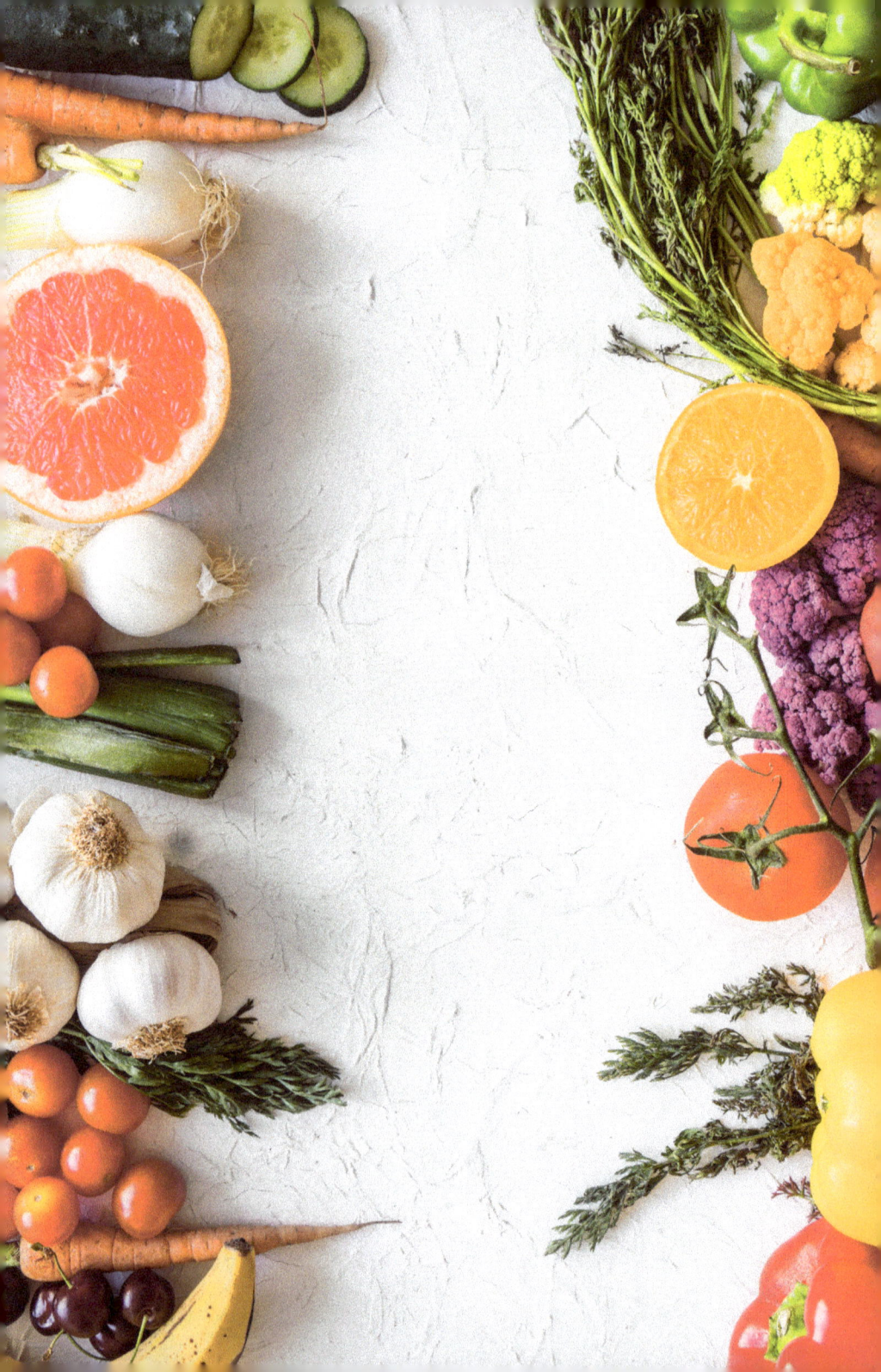

The philosophy of uncooked food

Food can be the chief source of trouble and, after many years of careful study and experimenting, experts are telling us that uncooked or raw food is the answer to our problems. It's a well-known fact that consuming too many grains, gluten and stodgy food will take your vitality away. Life food is logical. If you want to feel alive, eat live, wholesome food.

First of all, body, mind and spirit are absolutely interdependent, and if we recognise this fact we are a lot closer to understanding that correct nutrition for the body will help the mind and spirit to develop.

Since the human body is composed of certain chemicals, accurately proportioned, and since food is intended for the replacement of worn-out body cells, it logically follows that the food should contain the correct chemicals, properly combined, for that purpose. We have had an era of improving upon nature until we can scarcely tell just what is left of the original food when it reaches our tables.

Wheat and rice now have the most valuable parts polished off the exterior, corn has the oil and the heart removed from the interior, and we eat whatever the manufacturer has seen fit to leave for us. There is great inspiration for us to eat food as nature has grown it. If we cook spinach, we completely change the chemistry of that vegetable until it is doubtful if it is even ordinarily wholesome. We have destroyed the iron content and boiled the life out of the food. Think about that for just a moment before you read on. Ironically, preparation of a traditional cooked meal takes many hours of exacting toil in a heated temperature, and the weary cook sees the product of hours of work vanish in half an hour. If he or she wonders what the use of it all is, the honest answer is chiefly to create painful disturbances in the interior departments of the various members of the family and, consequently, to invite medical bills and more 'inefficiency' in the individual victims of cooked food.

> *"TELL ME WHAT A MAN OR WOMAN EATS AND I WILL TELL YOU WHAT MANNER A MAN OR WOMAN THEY ARE!"*

You should understand that the adoption of an uncooked diet does not mean a constant sacrifice of all the great foods to which you have been accustomed. A taste for fresh and delicious fruits, vegetables, cereals and nuts is readily acquired, and a cleaner palate soon discovers a delicacy and sweetness in raw foods that the highly seasoned and cookery-disguised foods never had.

Raw food does not produce disease, because it does not decay or ferment in the alimentary canals (or digestive tract). It does not produce toxic elements and therefore has true remedial value for curing disease by supplying the proper food elements in organic form.

Between 50,000 and 100,000 different chemicals go into the making and running of the human body. Nutritional science has so far isolated and identified some 17 vitamins and cofactors, 24 minerals, and 8-10 amino acids as being essential to the health and reproductive abilities of the human body. These essential nutrients need each other.

Cooking and other forms of processing interfere with this complexity and destroy much of this structural balance.

A HIGH RAW DIET...WHAT DOES IT OFFER?

A high raw diet offers two precious things:

1. Greater resistance to illness and ageing

2. Greater aliveness and vitality.

Resistance to illness and ageing:

Let us look closely at this resistance to illness and ageing. Everyone wants to live a long and healthy life. No one wants to look like a dried prune either. Read and re-read the following slowly.

So far, the most promising anti-ageing substances found in food are the antioxidants, nutrients such as vitamin A, C, E, and some of the B vitamins, the trace element selenium, the sulphur containing amino acids, and certain food preservatives such as BHT (butylated hydroxytoluene). These substances help to prevent the destructive oxidation processes that break down a cell's genetic material, which is ageing on a cellular level. Leading researchers on ageing believe that adding some or all of these antioxidants to our diet in sufficient quantities can hold back many age-related changes and increase longevity too.

Raw foods sharpen up an organism's ability to distinguish what is natural (self) from 'other'. The special enzyme called superoxide dismutase discourages the formation of 'rogue' molecules called superoxides and free radicals. These molecules do serious oxidative damage to every part of the body.

Let us consider the changes that take place when we change to a raw food diet. Skin loses its slackness and puffiness and seems to cling to the bones better. The true shape of the face emerges where once it was obscured by excess water retention and poor circulation. Lines become softer. Eyes take on the brightness and clarity that you may recall you had in your youth.

When you eat most of your vegetables, fruits, seeds and nuts raw you do not need so many calories. Nor do you want to eat as much as you would on a 'normal' diet. This is because a high raw diet contains such a lot of fibre and does not overstimulate the digestive system and make you want to eat more and more. Have you ever noticed how you tend to overeat on cooked food more than you do on raw food? It is the body's way of telling you that you haven't nourished yourself correctly.

Aliveness and vitality:

Aliveness and vitality are just natural side effects of a high raw diet. You will experience less negative feelings, a sign that body chemistry is in balance and toxins are being eliminated.

Chronic fatigue, 'the modern civilisation terror', is attributable to a deficit of the minerals potassium and magnesium. Fresh green vegetables and sprouts (rich in chlorophyll and thus magnesium) are the foods to combat fatigue.

A raw food diet affects blood sugar levels. Hypoglycaemia (low levels of sugar in the blood) can be controlled by a high raw diet. Mood swings and other symptoms of hypoglycaemia will disappear before too long and other people around you will notice a change in you before you notice it yourself.

Think about it...every day we build and nourish our bodies in some manner. Logically, a sound healthy body cannot be built of poor material. If you have built your body year after year of poor material, we must not expect to rejuvenate ourselves quickly. There are no miracles in nature. Results of a lifetime of indulgence in cooked food can't be expected to be eradicated in just a few meals of natural foods. When making the change to natural or uncooked food, people who have existed (and that's really all they are doing) for years on devitalised foods sometimes complain of not feeling satisfied by their new diet. This is because their body cells are clamouring for the old stimulants – cooked foods – from which they were built. Such individuals usually do not realise that the artificial energy, which they experience for a time on the cooked foods diet, is due to a whipping or irritation of the nerves by the poisons with which the system is loaded.

In cleansing a dirty house, dust will arise and inconveniences must be endured. When you resolve to cleanse yourself after a long period of wrongdoing or living, it must be remembered that the eliminations that will occur are preliminary to the rebuilding process.

Perseverance will be rewarded with normal and healthy reactions. The cleansing period will be shortened if, in addition to natural food, sun and air baths, elimination of toxins through the skin, deep breathing and exercise are maintained. I will elaborate more on this in the following chapters.

It is not necessary to talk and think food until you become paranoid about what you put in your mouth. I believe it is better to go about the real business of living, knowing that the body will not intrude upon our attention with the usual burden of ills which mankind unnecessarily endures. We can go about our daily activities feeling our very best if we just go back to basics, if we study the water content theory which I will explain in the following chapter, and observe and respect the laws of nature and the needs of others.

THE 75% TO 25% RULE FOR LIFE

Most of us do not consider the composition of our food. I'm suggesting that we take responsibility for what we consume and reinforce our chances of a strong resistance to disease and fatigue.

Every day we must nourish our bodies. Some of us just eat for the sake of it, some take a little time to include a few pieces of fruit, while others ignore all logic and eat what's in front of them regardless of its nutritional benefit.

Take time now to learn a few rules that will save your life. Does that sound too dramatic? Well, if it does, I make no apology at all, for I'm assuming that you have invested in this book as you are looking for a fresh start based on sound advice and solutions. I know I can deliver that, but I need your cooperation and willingness to apply the following philosophy.

Each day we must try to have at least 75% of our food as water-content food. What is water-content food? Fresh fruit and vegetables and water. The remaining 25% can be concentrated. Concentrated foods are grains, seeds, nuts, dairy, eggs, fish and meat to name a few. Notice I said the word 'can'. Actually, you can function on just fruit and vegetables alone and function beautifully! Some people will have higher needs for more protein and even more calories, depending on their physical activity. This is a state of physical awareness that you will acquire if you haven't already!

Interestingly enough, high-water-content foods are also alkaline-forming in the body whereas concentrated foods are acid-forming. To understand acid and alkaline foods we must imagine them having an acidic or alkaline reaction in the body after digestion. This refers to the chemical nature of their ash residues, determined by whichever minerals assert their presence in the blood after catabolism, with a further factor in determination being the presence or absence of acid residues in the blood. The taste of food itself does not determine its acidity or alkalinity from a nutritional standpoint.

ALKALINE-FORMING FOODS – COLD ... YING

75%

Fruits, fresh vegetables, fresh sprouted foods, water

Having established which foods are acid and which are alkaline, you need to consider everything you consume for a while in terms of its water content, etc., until it becomes automatic. You will be virtually learning how to eat all over again. Unfortunately, relatives and friends will make it very hard for you to change your eating habits unless they are responsible enough to join in with you.

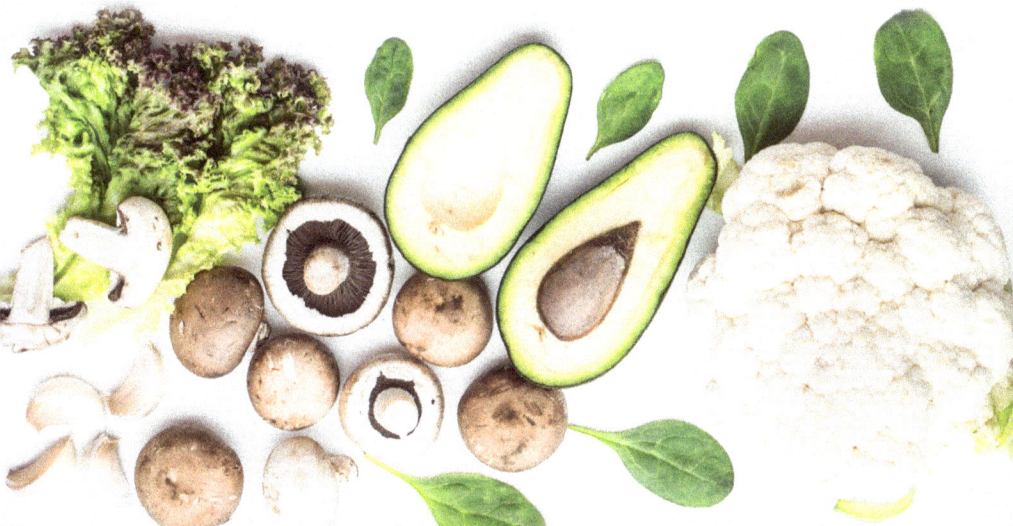

Fruits and vegetables are eliminating and cleansing foods – and are alkaline-forming. Starches and proteins are bodybuilders – and are acid-forming. You always want a more alkaline body. A too acidic condition breeds disease. There must always be a proper balance, but we all tend to eat not enough of the alkaline-forming eliminative fresh fruits and vegetables. Poisons move out of the body when raw fruits and vegetables are eaten.

If you've been feeling weak, check to see if you are getting enough of the body purifiers – fresh fruits and vegetables.

When buying or eating food always remember that the more processes a food has to go through before it gets to you, the quicker you should decide against buying and eating it. The more devitalised and processed foods you eliminate from your diet, the healthier you will be!

ACID-FORMING FOODS – HOT ... YANG

25%

Grains (rye, wheat, rice), **animal foods** *(meat, poultry and fish, with eggs only slightly acidic)*, **beans and lentils** *(unless they are sprouted)*, **nuts** *(especially peanuts and walnuts, and to a lesser extent, brazil nuts and hazelnuts. Almonds are very alkalising).*

Acid-producing foods are generally concentrated sources of protein and starch. They are foods whose residues contain more of the acid-producing minerals sulphur, phosphorus and chlorine than alkalising minerals such as calcium and magnesium. Other chemical producers of acidity are the organic acids such as oxalic and tannic. Beverages such as coffee, tea and cocoa are extremely acid-forming due to their high concentration of oxalic acid and, in tea, tannic acid. Pause for a moment and think of the acid-forming foods you have consumed the previous day. Were you tired? Were you aggressive? It is often the case that when you are particularly stressed out and grumpy, the whole feeling has become exasperated due to the diet being high in acid-forming foods.

Many fruits taste acidic, but this is physiological, not chemical. This acidity is due to the presence of a variety of organic acids in the fruits – citric acid, malic acid and tartaric acid. All of these are oxidised in catabolism, converting the fruit to alkaline in the process. The only acid not handled is oxalic acid, for the body finds this very difficult to absorb and seeks to neutralise it in the kidneys with the vital alkalising minerals calcium and magnesium. It is these two minerals, plus sodium, potassium and iron, which are major factors in determining whether a food is alkaline.

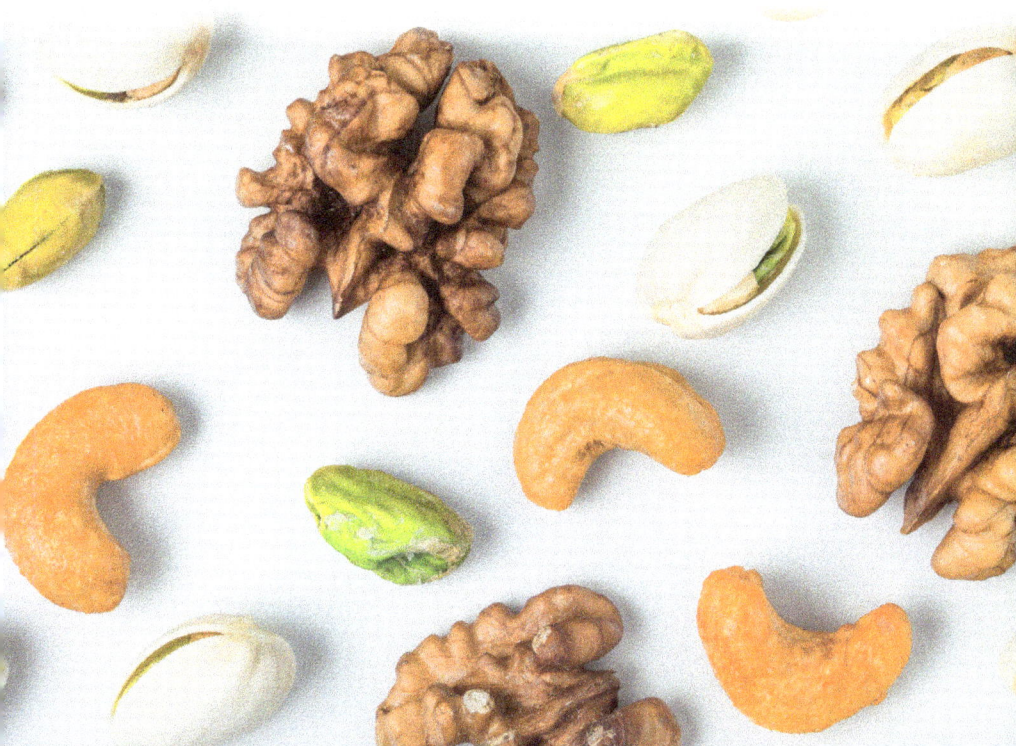

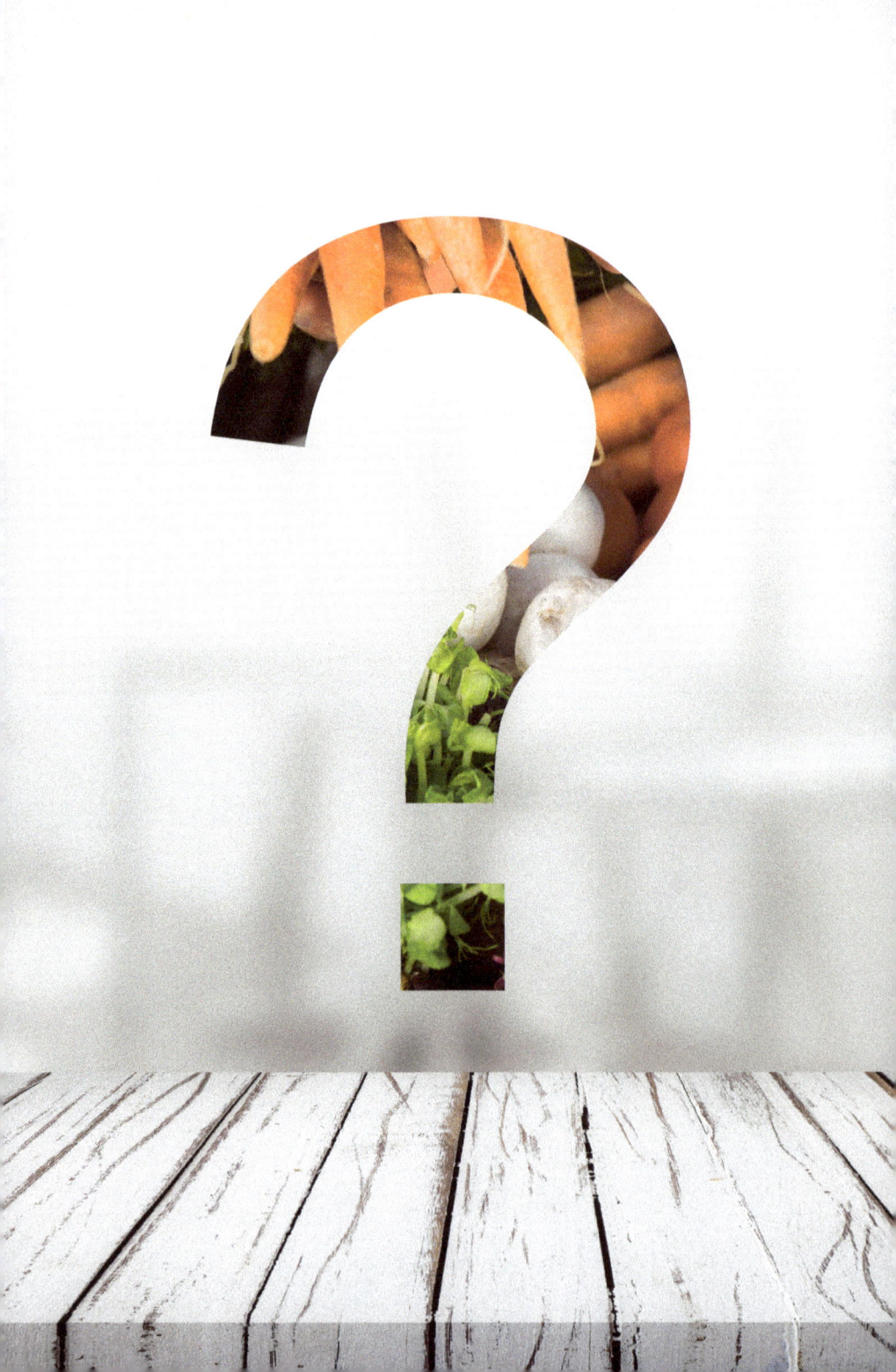

To cook or not to cook

Cooking food produces the most serious temptation to overeating. The smell of food being 'spoiled' in a fry pan seems to stimulate the appetite, yet food that is cooked or processed in any way must sacrifice much of its optimum nutrient content. Cooking food softens the food fibres so that less chewing is required; thus, less insalivation takes place. Both factors lead to overeating.

I'm not saying that cooked foods do not sustain life; in fact, you can function on cooked foods for quite some time, as you can see by the people around you. However, a diet too high in cooked foods can lead to slow but progressive degeneration of cells and tissues, and encourage early ageing and the development of degenerative diseases. Wouldn't it be exciting to think that we could regenerate and enhance health, as can happen on a high raw diet?

We know that cooking food destroys many essential nutrients. In fact, food processing and cooking, particularly at high temperatures, also brings about changes in the nature of food proteins, fats and fibre. This not only renders food constituents to be less health promoting to the body but may even make them harmful.

Vitamin C and B vitamins are water-soluble. As well as being very sensitive to heat, they leach out of food when it is soaked, blanched or boiled. Put a cabbage into cold water and bring it to boil and you destroy 75% of its vitamin C content. Cook fresh peas for longer than five minutes and there goes 30% of B1 (Thiamine). This may not mean anything to you until you learn a little more about vitamins and minerals later on this book.

When proteins are heated some amino acids become so 'denatured' that they are rendered useless. A protein is a chain of amino acids, some 20 of which are known in nature. Strung together in special sequences amino acids make up all the proteins there are, however only 8-10 of them appear to be essential for human nutrition, and our bodies need all of those almost all of the time.

Damaging proteins by cooking is not only wasteful but also obliges you to eat more to get the amino acids you need, which is risky in view of the links between high protein consumption, early ageing and the development of many degenerative diseases.

Heating fats to high temperatures changes the molecular structure of the fatty acids. In the heat processes involved in making margarine, cooking oil and countless convenience foods, manufacturers convert valuable 'cis' fatty acids, which the body needs and can make use of, into 'trans' fatty acids, which the body cannot use. This is why it is possible to eat a lot of fat but fail to get the fatty acids you need. If you must fry food, olive oil is probably the safest since it contains only four fatty acids, but it should never be heated to smoking point. I suggest you forget about frying food altogether and consider the wonderful alternatives.

The body recognises cooked food as a harmful invader and does its best to get rid of it. White blood cells flock to the intestines to deal with cooked food while the rest of the body is left undefended. This can put considerable strain on the immune system. Raw foods leave the white blood cells free for other tasks and save the body from defensive action, thereby strengthening its resistance.

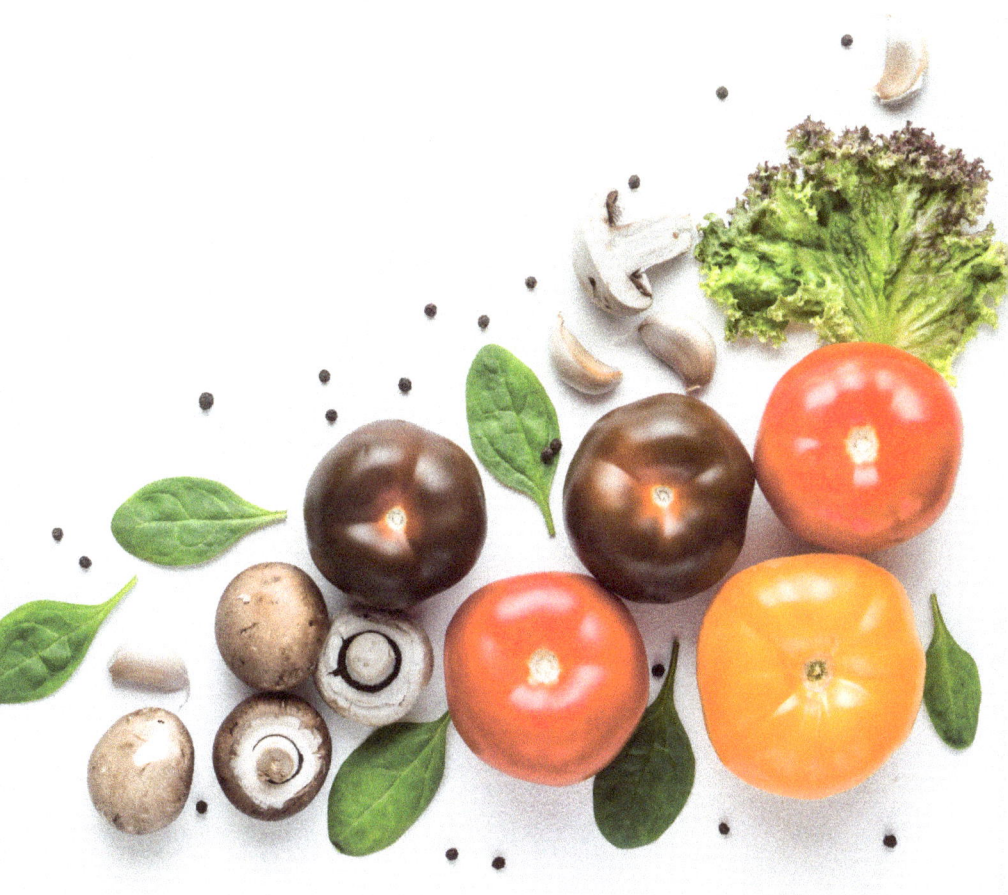

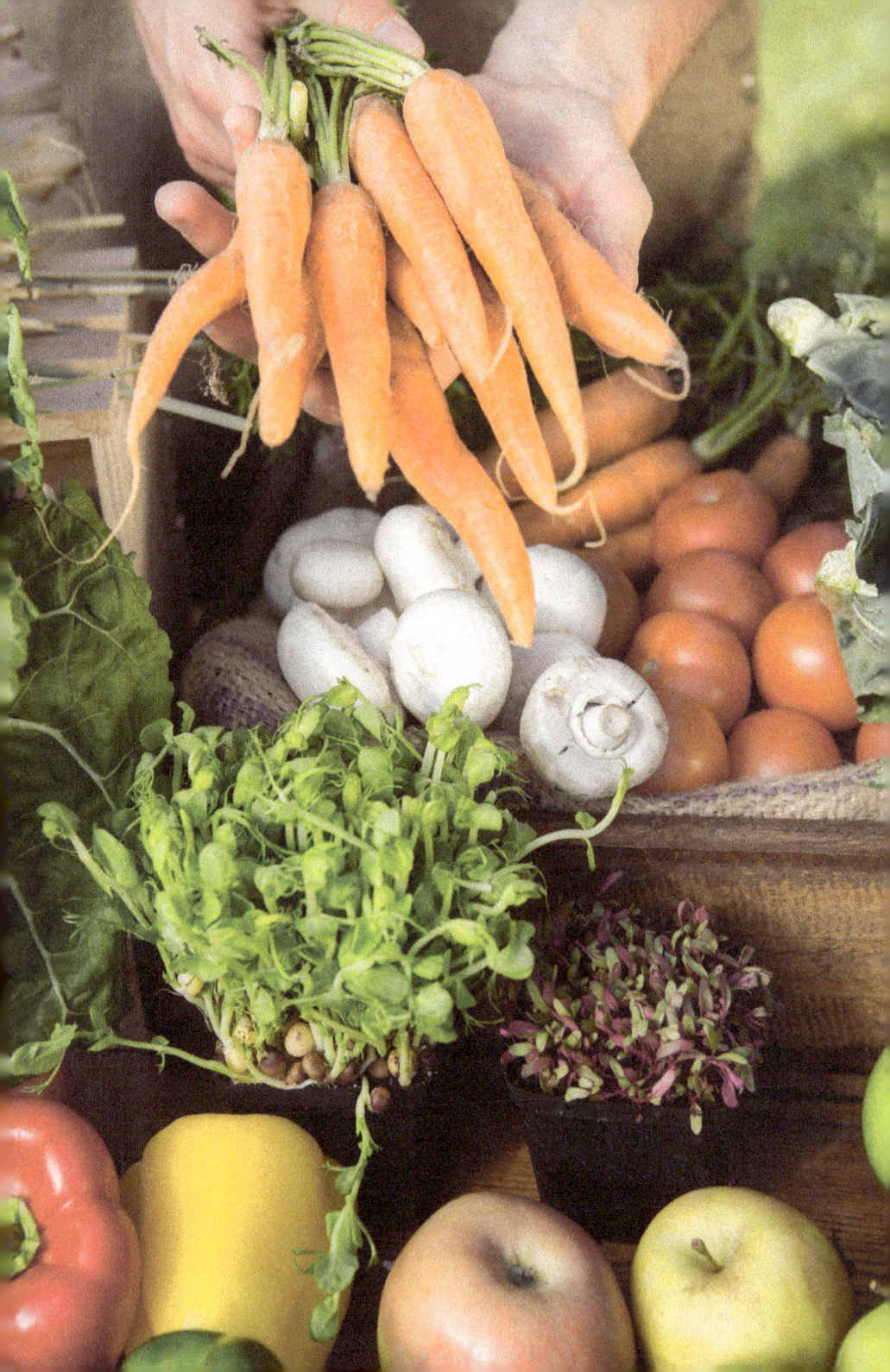

 # A way of eating

We all have to eat, don't we? No one knows your body and your energy levels better than you. Until you are ready to learn about and take responsibility for your own body, confusion will always linger when it comes to choosing your food. Take the time to observe your reactions to certain foods. Are you sleepy after you eat food with wheat as a dominant ingredient? Are you fuzzy in the head?

We are sick and overweight because we eat more refined food than we do natural, pure food. Fruits, vegetables, grains, nuts and seeds have the perfect balance of vitamins, minerals and digestive enzymes.

For early man the choices were simple. You ate what was in season. But now you have the choice of any kind of food at any time you want. Food travels thousands of kilometres over oceans and is often kept in cold storage, so by the time it gets to you it has a whole new vibration and may be another aggressive element that your body has to deal with rather than actually being good for you.

We are continually surrounded by too much food that is too easily accessible. I have learned a way of eating that is simple, balanced, and easy to understand...that is to *eat food as close as possible to the way it really is!*

THE 4 W'S – A WAY OF EATING

Before you eat anything consider the 4 W's:

1. WHAT: *Eat 75% high-water-content foods and 25% concentrated foods.*

2. WHY: *We must eat to nourish and live. So many of us eat because we have nothing better to do.*

3. WHERE: *Our surroundings and environment have a profound relationship to the way we digest our food and feel afterwards.*

4. WHEN: *We should eat when there is a decent rumble in the tummy and when you know you will have time to digest the food.*

The whole of this book deals with WHAT and WHY we eat, but before we go any further, it is important to discuss WHERE and WHEN a little further.

I believe we should have a quiet, peaceful environment to eat our food. There should be no outside distractions, like television or arguments that would cause us to forget about the action of eating, causing us to overeat or even fail to digest our food properly.

Perhaps the most important of the four W's is WHEN should you eat. Basically, two meals a day is plenty. I can just imagine what the average person would think of that but please let me explain further before you close the book. We must remember that digestion requires an incredible amount of energy. It is estimated that it takes as much energy to digest a poor combination of food as it does to run nearly a kilometre at your fastest speed.

In the Raw

In some people, poorly combined food and irregular body chemistry can lead to constant hunger and no feelings of satisfaction, no matter how much they have eaten. It occurs because your body cannot properly assimilate all the essential vitamins and minerals. It is vitally important properly functioning digestive enzymes regulate hormone function and the immune system itself, especially as our bodies age. We need to give our bodies time between meals to digest the food from the previous meal. I suggest your first meal should be fruit at around 11.00am–12.00pm.

Most of you are probably brainwashed into the idea that you should begin the day with a hearty breakfast. Well, I'm sure the local butcher or even cereal manufacturer would love you to continue to think that way, as it will keep them in business longer and your life shorter!

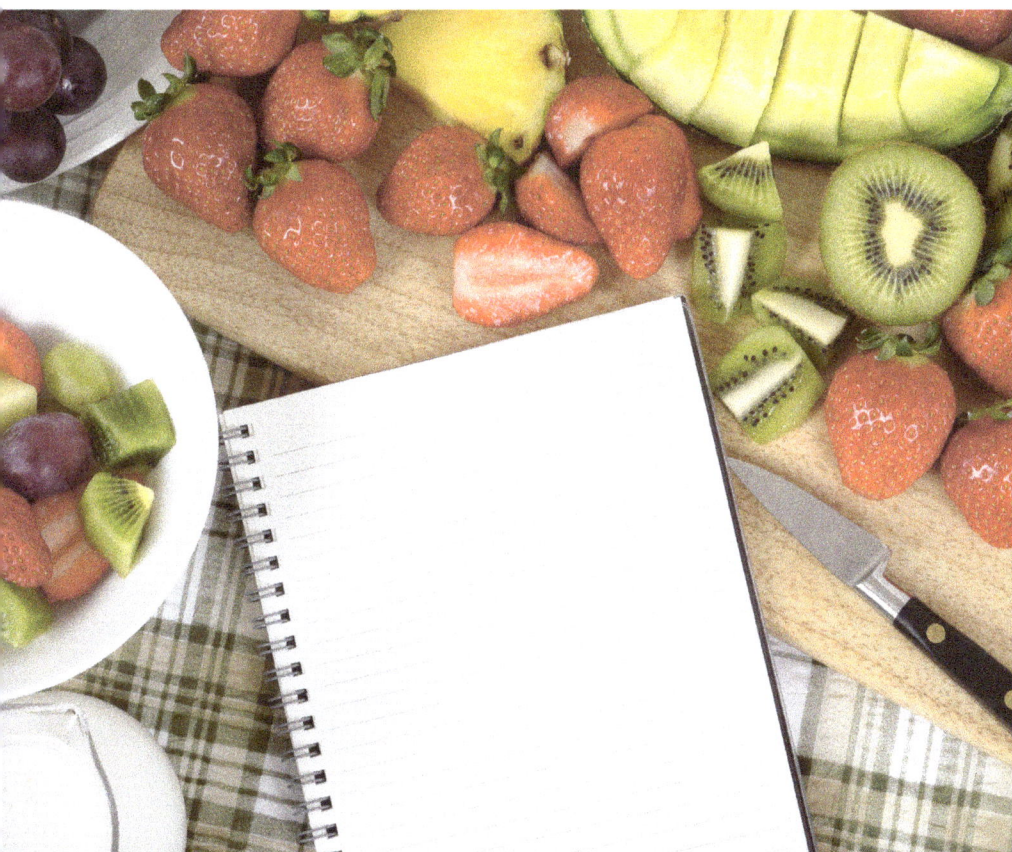

Forget the cereals, eggs and bacon, and give yourself a break. Start your day without digestive overload and feel the difference. Make up a fruit platter and take it to work or grab a few pieces of fruit and munch them when you feel hungry.

The next meal should follow at about 6.00–7.00pm. This can be a meal of salad and nuts, etc. You may prefer to have a salad at lunchtime as well. That is fine. There are no rules here. We don't live in a perfect world, so we do not have to be perfect. There will be times when you will want to eat in between meals. That's fine, so long as it is a high-water-content food and that you do not overeat.

If you really need to have breakfast, have fruit juice or fruit, as you will digest this quickly enabling you to expend your energy on doing your work or playing or whatever. While I'm working I try not to eat anything until I'm finished. The food is a reward when I have put all my energy into the project at hand.

Try not to eat late at night or before going to bed. Remember your body wants to rest. Eating food before trying to sleep is like running a marathon after you have just completed another. Let your digestion rest and ensure a peaceful sleep. Remember, whatever you plan to eat will more than likely be there the next day. The end of the day is the danger zone for so many weight watchers because it is usually when resistance levels are at their lowest.

If you are not hungry then don't eat until you are. It's that simple!

Detoxification & the three-day clean up

Detoxification is not new, nor is it something that 'health cranks' carry out as some sort of ritual. *Detoxification is vital for a really healthy, happy individual.* There are certain potential discomforts, but they can definitely be minimised. You must remember that there will be a build-up of toxic waste in some of you that has been building up over the years. It is absolutely essential for the system to be cleansed so that energy can be freed up to be used in reducing weight and helping the body to function as it really should. The possible discomforts depend on how toxic your system is. Through fasting you will find out just how toxic you are, believe me.

The three-day clean up

So you know something is wrong. You seem to need more sleep than usual. You still wake up tired. Your moods are up and down. You are eating without control or thought. What you are eating is lacking in nutrition and water content. You feel depressed. Your stomach is bloated and you're putting on weight. To top it off you are under a lot of pressure and feeling stressed out.

The Three-Day Clean Up (3DCU) could be your salvation! The 3DCU is not an easy solution. It will work and you will come out of it feeling wonderful, although with a little discomfort and mental anguish along the way. But it will be worth every moment and even more valuable if you practice good eating habits thereafter. You can expect to experience bloating of the system due to the stirring up of accumulated toxic waste creating gas. You may experience headaches or body aches. You may feel suddenly tired or anxious. You may experience loose, runny stools (diarrhoea). Nausea is also quite common during detoxification and especially when you fast for the first time. *You may think fasting is crazy stuff and that you'll die if you miss out on lunch! I say you'll live longer if you reduce the meals you eat.*

Before it begins you must make some preparations that will minimise some of the nasty side effects. A week before, eliminate certain foods from your diet. This will likely reduce the discomfort you will feel with the upcoming change and create the headspace needed to continue looking after yourself and your eating habits. If you are not prepared to reduce or eliminate these foods then the cleanse could be more destructive than beneficial.

Foods to eliminate: Tea, coffee, chocolate, alcohol, sugar (all), dairy, meat, fish, eggs, spices, onion, pasta and cakes.

Foods to increase: Fruit, vegetables, simple grains like millet and rice and (for energy) dried fruit and nuts.

WARNING during pregnancy and nursing

Pregnant women and nursing mothers should not fast at all. Wait for six months after having a baby before fasting. For those with a serious illness, such as diabetes, liver or kidney disease, tuberculosis, hypoglycaemia or heart problems a doctor should be consulted before you begin a fast or any sort of detoxification. Anyone who is extremely underweight would be wise to seek advice from a professional. Underweight people can still cleanse themselves on fruit and vegetable juices.

Day one

On the first day you fast. Yep, you got it, you don't eat all day! Naturally this is the day when you have nothing major planned. As you become more experienced with fasting, you will be able to go out and even go to work, but for your first attempt I recommend you stay home and rest!

The night before starting the 3DCU you should not eat anything after 8.00pm. You will wake up on the morning of day one and drink two glasses of water. If you wish you can exercise lightly. Just go for a quiet walk and think about the day ahead. Continue to drink water all day and rest when you are feeling hungry. If you have a family and usually prepare their meals, then organise their meals the day before.

To fast means to abstain from all foods and drink only water. When you fast, the body is free to do the thing it does best, which is a natural self-healing and cleansing process. When you are not filling the body with food for a period of time, all the energy that is usually used to digest, assimilate and metabolise is now spent in purifying the body. This is also a time of new cell growth even though you are not feeding the body. We have within us plenty of nourishment to sustain us well beyond a three-day fast. You may be relieved to know that I'm not suggesting you go on a three-day fast as part of this program.

Fasting eliminates poisons from the system very efficiently; when you feel a minor illness coming on, a fast can sometimes prevent its development by allowing the body to concentrate on the self-healing and cleansing process. Many of us are usually sitting in the waiting room of a doctor's clinic before we even consider a fast as a cure, *however please consider this option as it's cheaper and better for you. Nature is slower than the doctor and medications, but far better for you in the long run.*

If you fast regularly you will find that you are less susceptible to colds, flu, sinus problems, and various allergic reactions. Fasting repairs a crippled digestive tract. Your stomach will begin to shrink in size, making it easier for you to control the amount of food you eat. Fasting re-educates your taste buds, stopping you from craving junk.

If you are awake at 7.30am, then by 10.00am you may experience some hunger pangs. Hunger pangs are messages from the stomach that there simply is not enough activity, not (as some would believe) that you will die if you don't eat something! Drink water when you feel those pangs. Around 4.00–5.00pm you may be feeling really hungry or you may have a very nasty headache, so lie down, relax and drink some more water. Hang in there until it's time to go to bed. You may not be tired but try to sleep. In the morning you will have your reward. You will have survived the first day and notice that you are still alive. Some people sleep soundly, others just dream, toss, turn and wake early. You can expect to feel a little weak and maybe even sick. That is part of toxic elimination. If you don't feel this way at all, good! You probably were not all that toxic to begin with. Sometimes this can be an illusion, as it may take several days of fasting before the real nasties come out. For more information, see Fasting section in this book.

Day two

Okay, so you are awake and ready for day two. The taste of a freshly squeezed watermelon juice should be quite something. On this second day we are going to enjoy fruit juice all day. If you can handle it, I would stick to two kinds of fruit only.

For your first 3DCU, stick to watermelon, grapes or apples. These are good cleansing fruits and will give you the energy to get through this second day.

Juices are the next best thing to the whole food, being merely a liquid extract of the whole food. They supply us with vital building blocks for cell regeneration; a true longevity food.

Freshly squeezed juices are the preferred beverages that can help you lose weight and feel great. I'm not talking about juices you buy in bottles from the local supermarket; they are poor substitutes for the real thing and in many cases will only add to the toxic overload due to the preservatives that are added to the liquid. Anything that has a long shelf life is suspect in my opinion.

Remember to drink your juice slowly, mixing the juice with your saliva. Gulped or consumed too rapidly, the juice may upset the blood sugar level.

On this second day you will be feeling pretty happy with yourself for having made it through the first day. Exercise lightly and increase the juice intake as you see fit. Take some deep breaths if you feel nauseated and lie down for a while. If you don't feel like drinking juice, then don't. You don't have to force food down your system for the sake of it. That is what causes so many problems in the first place.

Anne Clark

Before you go to bed that night, drink a warm glass of water with lemon juice. This will help with any bad breath that may have developed and helps with internal cleansing. Hopefully you would have experienced several bowel movements by now; if not the warm water and lemon juice could be a solution to that problem. Keep in mind that any time you alter your eating habits, your body has to adjust to that change and in so doing can initially leave you feeling out of sorts. You are witnessing the cleansing process and health in action.

The total elimination of all toxicity from your body can take months or years, but within days you will be feeling enormously more energetic and vibrant.

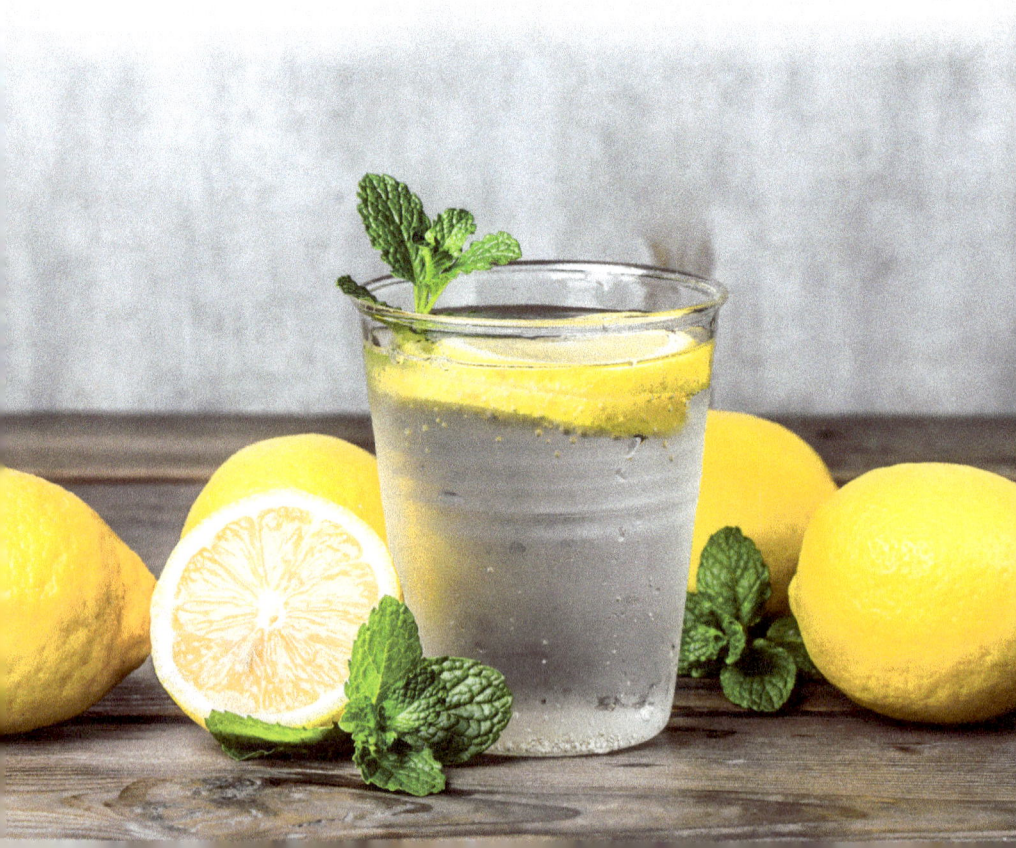

Day three

By the third day you are ready for some solid fruit. No vegetables at all today. We do not want to introduce the starch of the vegetable so soon to a cleansed system. We want to encourage further cleansing to continue by the consumption of fruit.

Fruit is the one food that the human species is biologically adapted to. It requires less energy to be digested than any other food. Everything consumed by the human body must eventually be broken down and transformed into glucose, fructose, glycerine, amino acids and fatty acids. The brain cannot function on anything but glucose (sugar). Fruit is glucose in the body. Other foods spend from one to four hours in the stomach, provided the food eaten has been properly combined. Fruits are pre-digested. They pass through the stomach in 20 to 30 minutes. Fruits break down and release nutrients in the intestines. The energy conserved by not having to be broken down in the stomach is considerable. This energy is automatically redirected to cleanse the body of toxic waste, which ultimately will help to reduce weight.

Fruit should never be eaten with or immediately following other food. It should never be cooked, canned, or consumed in pies, pastry, etc. Cooking destroys its potential cleansing value. The body is only capable of utilising fruit in its natural state. So today enjoy fruit in its whole state. The body is adjusting now to a little more effort with digestion and we should notice an energy lift.

REMEMBER...A WHOLE FOOD IS ALWAYS BETTER THAN ONE THAT HAS BEEN FRAGMENTED.

Anne Clark

I always like to have some pineapple or pawpaw on the third day. The flavours are so special and you will find your tastes have become even more sensitive due to the initial fast on day one.

By the time the third day is over you will feel the benefits of the 3DCU. On the following morning (day four), try to consume only fruit until midday. You may like to have a salad for lunch consisting of grated carrot and beetroot (see recipes) or more fruit.

Your body will tell you what it wants! Avoid cooked or processed foods for the next few days or the rest of your life if you wish.

The next time you carry out a detoxification program you will be more experienced. Provided you continue to observe the high-water-content theory – *75% water-content and 25% concentrated – you may not even need to do another 3DCU!*

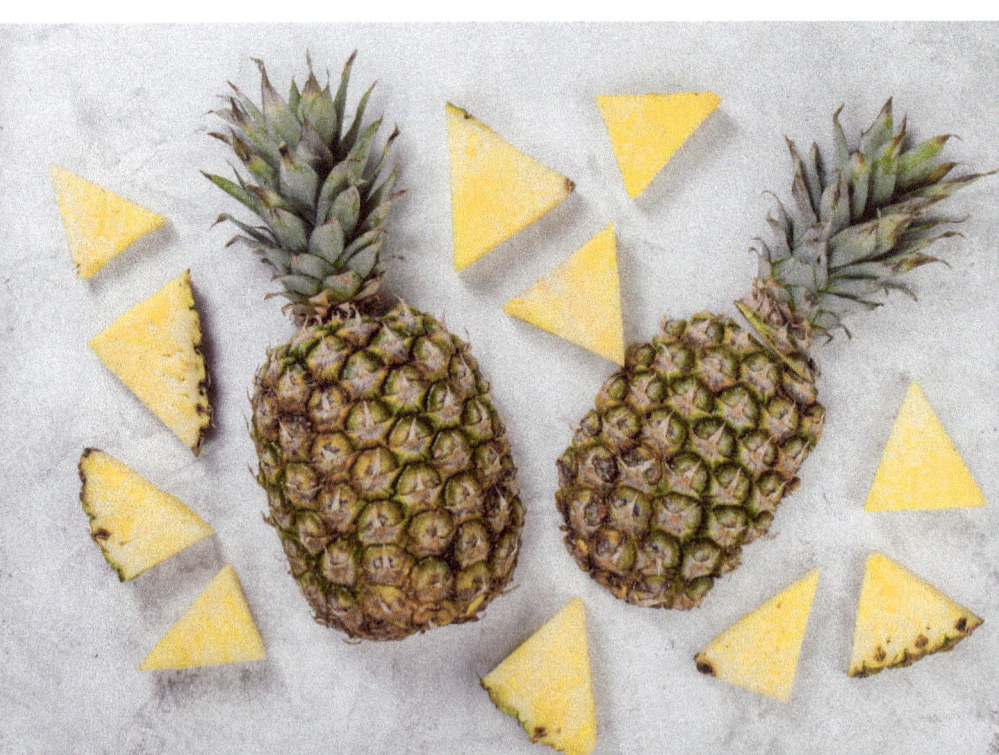

Symptoms of toxic elimination

Generally, as fasting begins to loosen the toxins in the body, there are many symptoms that give you an indication of what is going on inside of you. These signs of toxic elimination leave when the poisons are gone.

Headaches are common during fasting, especially if you are new to fasting and have mistreated your body with processed food or if you regularly have caffeine drinks like coffee, tea or soft drinks. Disturbed sleep, restlessness, and strange or bad dreams sometimes occur during a fast. Generally, you don't require as much sleep to feel rested during a fast because your body isn't exhausted trying to digest all the food. Chills are common. It's okay in summer to feel cool, but if you feel chilled in the winter, don't hesitate to have a cup of warm water and wear extra clothing. Clogged sinuses, phlegm or a stuffy nose can all occur and are indicators of toxic poisons in the system and are signs that the body is trying to rid itself of them.

After the 3DCU, you will be so much stronger and your resistance to illness will be even greater. Take time to fill out the following chart as your record for future detoxification attempts.

Please note: The author welcomes the results of your 3DCU.

Please send this chart to:

anne@anneclark.com.au

Three-day clean up chart

Name:_____

Email:_____

Address:_____

DAY ONE

Record your feelings, level of discomfort and other comments_____

_____

DAY TWO

Please circle one or all of the juices consumed below:

Watermelon   Apple   Grape

Comments:_____

_____

Did you experience a bowel movement? _____

DAY THREE

List the fruits you ate on this day:_____

_____

Comments:_____

_____

In the Raw

OVERALL PROGRAM

Food cravings while on this program?_____

_____

Chart returned (Yes/No)? _____

Preferred phone number:_____

This chart is your record of how you coped while taking part in the 3DCU. I would love to know how you felt and I would appreciate any comments that would help me to determine how effective the detoxification was for you personally. Thank you.

Anne Clark

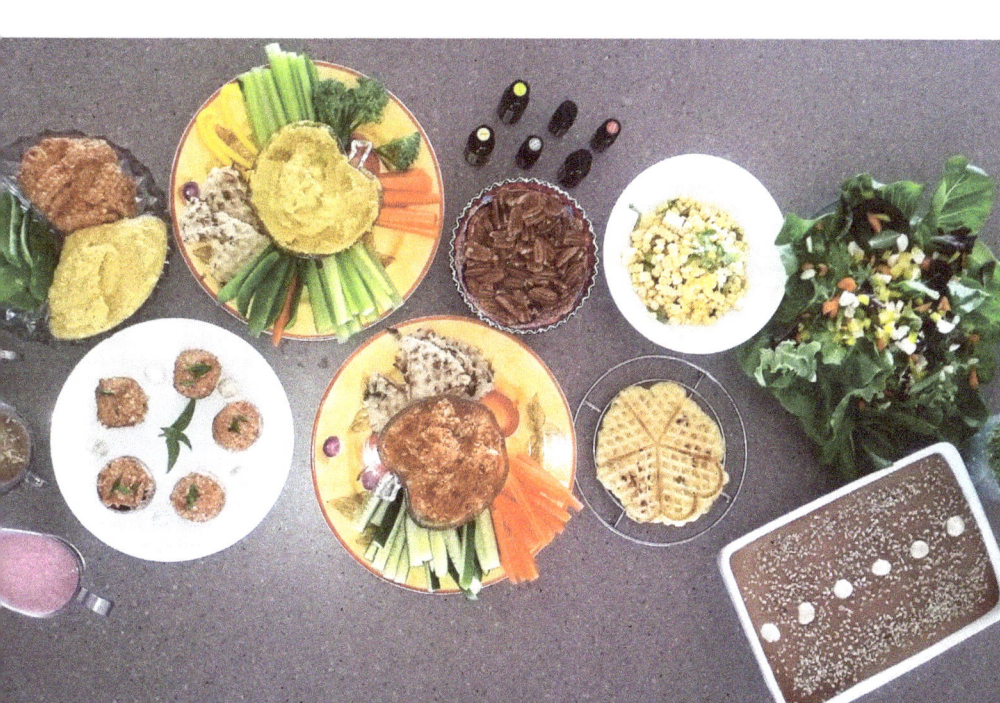

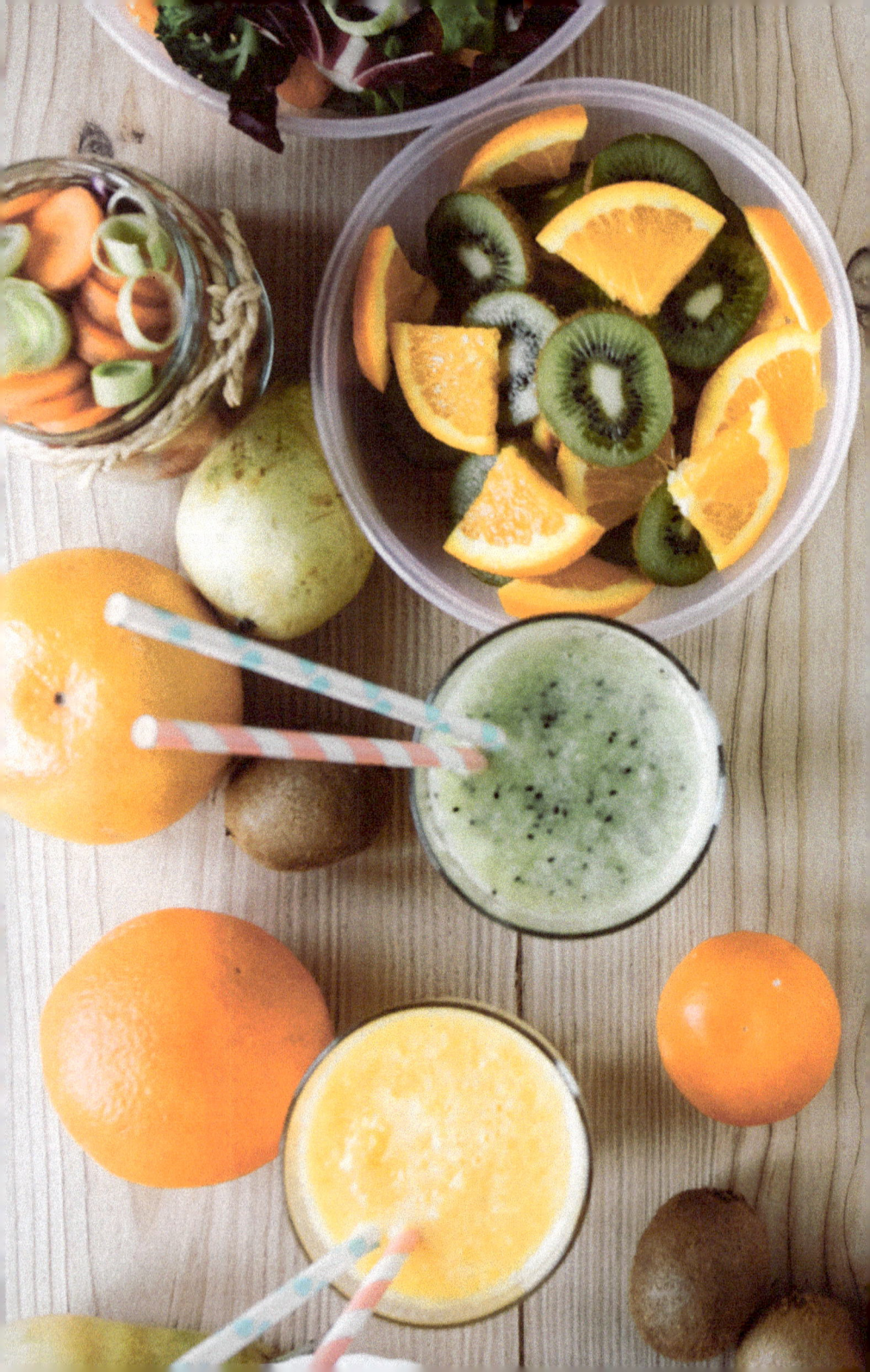

 # Vitamins and minerals

To me, it is pointless learning about vitamins and minerals, until we are prepared to remember what they are and how we can utilise them through our foods.

Supplementation with tablets, capsules or powders should not be necessary if we observe the 75% to 25% rule discussed in previous pages. There is some merit to taking supplements, but you must research the supplements beforehand and read the labels on containers thoroughly to be sure you are getting what you have paid for. While we are on the subject of paying, many people would do well to spend their money on more nutritious fruit and vegetables, which would reduce the need to spend money on supplementation in the first place.

WHAT ARE VITAMINS AND MINERALS?

Quite simply, **vitamins** are organic substances necessary for life. Vitamins are essential for the normal functioning of our bodies and, except for a few, cannot be manufactured or synthesised by our bodies. They are necessary for growth, vitality and general wellbeing.

Minerals are chemical compounds that form the essential structure and assist in the physiological functioning of the body. A good example of this would be to look closely at calcium. The basic hardness of bones and teeth is attributable to the salt form of adequate calcium stores.

If we wish to heal ourselves in terms of health, we can learn to increase or decrease our consumption of certain foods to treat various minor deficiencies or disease. If you feel you are coming down with a cold, you can either fast or increase your vitamin C (ascorbic acid) and vitamin P (bioflavonoids) foods. If you are constantly getting ulcers in the mouth, you are probably eating too many acid-forming foods, under stress and in need of more B vitamins. There are even foods to incorporate into your diet that will help your hair and skin to look their best. Below is a list of vitamins and minerals, but further reading is advised on the subject.

VITAMINS

Vitamin A – Retinol

Vitamin A is a fat-soluble vitamin. It enters the body in two different forms:

1. The fat of the animal (also contains toxic factors – cholesterol of the animal).

2. Plant foods, as carotene, the red or yellow colour of fruits and vegetables. Carotene is also found in green vegetables.

The most obvious indication of a vitamin A deficiency is night blindness. Acne, boils, skin ulcers, emphysema, chronic nephritis and skin abnormalities can be treated with vitamin A. This vitamin is known to directly support all cellular growth, especially the eyes, the organs, outer tissues of the body (skin, hair and gums), and the bones and teeth.

This is probably the most sensitive vitamin in terms of minor toxicity from overdosage due to its ease of internal storage. For this reason, care should be taken. If too much is ingested, the liver will overflow and induce a yellowness in the skin and the eyes with a possible feeling of nausea.

Best food sources of carotene are: parsley, carrots, silverbeet, yellow sweet potatoes, and all green, yellow and red fruits and vegetables. Best sources of retinol are: cod liver oil, animal livers, butter, egg yolk, margarine, and milk and its products (care must be taken with these items in the diet; I do not recommend them).

Vitamin B – Complex Group

This group of water-soluble compounds is generally found to occur in similar food sources. They are synergistic, being more potent together than when used separately. They all react differently to heat and light.

Vitamin B1 – Thamine

Thiamine cannot be stored in the body to any degree and must be taken daily through one's food. If you are constantly depressed, anxious, stressed out, worrying about nothing, experiencing tired muscles and heart, and often under the influence of alcohol, you may consider taking a B-complex vitamin with adequate amounts of thiamine.

Best whole food sources are: sunflower seed kernels, nuts, soya beans and whole grains. Soya milk, soya grits and soya flour are also highly beneficial sources. Meats, seafoods, dairy products, eggs and commercial cereals are not as high in thiamine as the various corporations behind these products would have you believe.

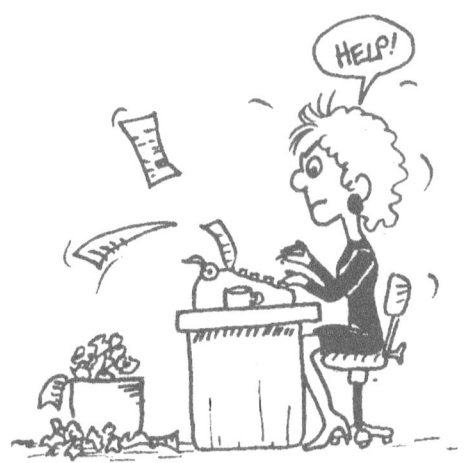

Vitamin B2 – Riboflavin

As with thiamine, daily food intake of riboflavin is essential. Consider those recurring, mouth, lip and tongue sores, soreness around the eyes, poor skin tone, weak nails and dull hair, and how they could possibly relate to a deficiency of riboflavin.

By increasing the same food sources as thiamine with the addition of parsley, you could protect yourself from the above problems. Riboflavin aids in growth and reproduction, and in megadoses is beneficial in overcoming an addiction to sugar, but then so is an all-raw diet! Possibly the two are related.

Vitamin B3 – Niacin/Niacinamide

There are two vitamins within B3 – nicotinic acid and nicotinamide (a nitrogenous alkaline compound). Their common names are niacin and niacin amide. Vitamin B3 is stable when exposed to heat, oxygen, and light. It is a vulnerable vitamin; in nature both forms of B3 are often bound to other nutrients, rendering them somewhat difficult to absorb in the body. B3 is easily leached out by water, especially boiling water. If you drink alcohol, take sleeping tablets, estrogen or sulphur drugs, and consume processed foods, you are probably deficient of this vitamin.

B3 is used in the treatment of schizophrenia and the pain and physical deterioration caused by arthritis and rheumatism. B3 has also been used to treat Pellagra, which is characterised by dermatitis with light-sensitive inflammations on the skin, plus diarrhoea, depression and, on occasion, psychotic disorders indicated by mental confusion.

The 'junk-food freak' would do well to consider a B3 supplement or *increase their consumption of peanuts (raw), mushrooms and dried fruits. Whole wheat, buckwheat, unpolished rice and corn are also suitable sources.* Next time you are having trouble concentrating, feeling apprehensive, anxious or worried, or suffering from cold hands or feet, buy some raisins or raw nuts and make a 'Brain Smoothie' (see recipe later in this book) and relax a little!

B3 has been recognised as a vital coenzyme in fat metabolism within the body, where it aids in the control of triglyceride and cholesterol levels. It also assists in relieving small painful mouth ulcers and halitosis (bad breath from indigestion). It is also a therapeutic aid to sufferers of senility. So, if you are becoming somewhat ancient, increase your B3 foods and keep your mind young.

Vitamin B5 – Pantothenic Acid

Once again, cooking destroys the positive effects of B5. The presence of caffeine (found in tea as well as coffee) also induces dietary losses of B5. It is a general growth, repair and maintenance vitamin, which helps to combat stress, allergies, constipation and transmittable illnesses.

Failure of the body's autoimmune system to produce sufficient antibodies can also be traced to inadequate vitamin B5, as can nerve degeneration, resulting in muscle weaknesses, often indicated by pins and needles in the body's extremities. Loss of memory and greying hair can both benefit from B5 in conjunction with PABA (Para-aminobenzoic acid) and Choline.

B5 is found in much the same foods as previous B vitamins as well as in dietary yeasts, nuts, seeds, mushrooms, soya beans, oatmeal, broccoli and avocados. The richest source is royal jelly. As every cell of the body benefits from B5, both before and after birth, pregnant women would do well to increase their intake of all the B vitamins to ensure a healthy baby and their own wellbeing.

Vitamin B6 – Pyridoxine

B6 is one of the most significant of the B-group for nutrition and therapeutic usefulness. Pyridoxine is destroyed by boiling water, food processing, and refined by alcohol and certain drugs. Estrogen is one of the most destructive. Women on the oral contraceptive pill would be on the high deficiency list. Kidney disorders and stones, dry or oily skin, autism and anaemia, nervousness, irritability, premenstrual tension, acne, stress, dandruff, aggressiveness, inflamed hands, dry and cracked heels, numbness or cramps in the arms or legs and hypoglycaemia can all be traced to a B6 deficiency.

B6 is very effective in alleviating nausea and combating morning sickness during pregnancy. While we are on morning sickness, this is really a sickness of the 20th century, as most women on pure, raw foods, do not experience morning sickness at all. The more protein-rich foods eaten, the more B6 the body demands. Caffeine foods, animal foods and seafoods really keep B6 busy. When combined with apple cider vinegar, kelp and lecithin it helps to control weight and the associated problems. It is helpful during pregnancy when fevers occur, where it should be combined with vitamin C for maximum benefit. B6 is found in similar foods as previous B vitamins.

Best natural sources are: dietary yeast, sunflower seed kernels, beans, wheat germ, lentils, buckwheat, brown rice, bananas, hazel nuts and avocados. Other rich sources are seafoods and organ meats.

Vitamin B12 – Cyanocobalamin

This vitamin influences fat metabolism. It is the only vitamin known to contain essential minerals – phosphorus and cobalt – as part of its structure.

Its security rests on the B12 produced in one's body. The stomach secretes a substance called 'intrinsic factor', which transports the vitamin B12 created by the bacterial flora in our intestines. Some authorities state that humans, unlike animals, cannot synthesise B12 in their liver, implying that vegetarians will be deficient in this vitamin if they do not take B12 supplements. Let me say for starters that we humans only need minute amounts of B12. The vitamin is found in plants in very small amounts and putrefaction hampers the secretion of the intrinsic factor in the stomach and retards production of B12. Vegetarians, therefore, are less likely to develop a B12 deficiency than meat eaters.

Let common sense prevail as you consider the animals whose meat you eat. Where do those animals get their B12?

The most important role of vitamin B12 is in overcoming pernicious anaemia. Symptoms include lethargy, impatience, incipient memory loss, etc. Before you say to yourself, "That's me", these symptoms are generally related to all B vitamins. It is known for its essential role in the development and regeneration of red blood cells, the correct metabolising of major nutrients, which helps to promote normal growth, increasing appetite of the young, energy, nourishing the nervous system, improving brain functioning and mental balance.

Most authorities insist that only animal foods possess adequate B12, but experience has shown the opposite to be true. Most vegetarians not only have a suitable blood count, but also have a lower than average blood pressure.

It could be that the human body can actually synthesise its own B12 in the liver with the aid of balanced food nutrients from plant foods. It is not surprising that, with a healthy body, plant foods known to be rich in B-complex vitamins are not devoid of minimal B12 plus cobalt to assist the body in synthesising additional quantities if needed.

Food sources are: most plant foods already listed for the previous vitamins, but those of special benefit are the whole grains, alfalfa sprouts and other green vegetables.

Vitamin B13 – Orotic Acid

This vitamin is known to have similar characteristics to other B vitamins in so far as its water solubility is concerned, and it is also known to assist in the metabolising of vitamin B12 and folic acid. Its main use is to help with better absorption of essential minerals, by combining with them chemically to form salts such as calcium orotate, magnesium orotate, etc.; especially beneficial whenever calcium and magnesium are required by the body.

Food sources are: whey liquid and powder, as well as root vegetables.

Vitamin B15 – Pangamic Acid

Like B13, little research has been undertaken on this vitamin. B15 works like vitamin E, in that it acts as an antioxidant. Exposure to sunlight and boiling water will greatly diminish the usefulness of B15.

It is known to improve heart conditions by working to overcome atherosclerosis of the coronary blood vessels and other cardiovascular diseases. It aids in the recovery from stress, exercise and fatigue. It also has the capability of neutralising the addiction to alcohol as well as contributing towards an increased life span.

Best food sources are: rice bran, apricot kernels, brewer's yeast, whole grains, all seeds, especially pumpkin seeds (pepitas) and most of the usual B-complex foods.

Vitamn B17 – Laetrile

The anti-cancer nutrient. Some practitioners consider that in large doses B17 can greatly assist a cancer sufferer to remit the disease, so long as he or she undertakes a vegetarian, raw food diet.

Food sources high in B17 are: wild blackberry, elderberry, seeds of deciduous fruit trees, mung beans, bitter almonds, macadamia nuts, bamboo and alfalfa sprouts. Slightly lower food sources are other berry fruits, including currants, as well as quince, buckwheat, linseed, millet, kidney beans, lentils and lima beans. It is the only B vitamin not found in brewer's yeast.

Biotin – Coenzyme

Biotin is essential for the normal metabolism of protein and fat. It is found in every living cell in minute amounts and is metabolically related to pantothenic acid and folic acid. Avidin is a proteinaceous compound that bonds with biotin to form a non-absorbable food, which could explain why so many people are found to be allergic to eggs. To avoid a loss factor of Avidin, eggs should be eaten raw, and the yolks must be separated from the whites and the whites avoided.

Extreme exhaustion, drowsiness, muscle pain and anorexia are just some of the conditions indicating a lack of biotin. Biotin alleviates dermatitis, eczema and loss of body weight, and assists in the maintenance of hair by keeping it in its natural colour, rather than greying, and helping to avoid baldness, a cause of which being a deficiency of nourishment to the scalp, facilitated by adequate nutrients and massage.

Food sources are: brewer's yeast, soya beans and their products (Textured vegetable protein), soya flour, soya grits, soy milk), rice bran and brown rice, egg yolk, nuts, whole grains, peas, cauliflower, mushrooms, wheat bran and lentils. Biotin is also available from animal foods like liver, fish and chicken. Once again, I do not recommend animal sources.

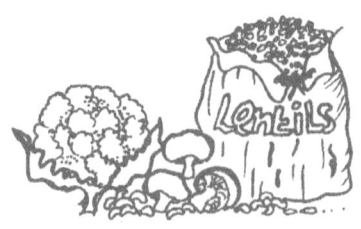

Choline

Choline can be made in the human gastrointestinal tract if not attendant in foods. It is a vital constituent of lecithin, a fat emulsifier. Poor memory, which sometimes leads to possible senility or Alzheimer's disease (in older people), is often a symptom of deficiency of choline.

As a component of lecithin, Choline (together with inositol) works to utilise fats and cholesterol, so that the fat can provide energy and the cholesterol is deterred from settling against the arterial wall or in the gall bladder. Many cases of nervousness and nervous twitching or fidgeting have been overcome by choline increase.

Premature greying of the hair and vitiligo, the skin disease, can be remedied by daily doses of choline in most cases.

Fortunately, availability of choline from the diet is widespread and abundant. Sources include: lecithin, egg yolk, wheatgerm, soya beans, black eye beans, brewer's yeast, chickpeas, lentils, split peas, brown rice and other whole grains, plus peanuts. Vegetables are also very valuable sources of choline. Only liver, ham and veal, amongst the meats, come within the high choline group, although they are not recommended as part of a good diet.

Folic Acid

Folic acid is important in the body's production of the nucleic acids (RNA and DNA) and is essential for the body's cellular mitosis (division and replacement). Too many medicinal or addictive drugs disrupt absorption.

Folic acid can be destroyed by being stored, or those foods containing it being stored, in open, unprotected conditions for extended periods, even at room temperature. Like other B vitamins it is heat and light sensitive.

Alcoholics would certainly be deficient in this vitamin as would drug addicts. Not only do women on the oral contraceptive pill need increased folic acid, but so do pregnant women. The unborn child demands a high quantity of folic acid. Unless she has been on a natural foods diet, supplementation will be advised. For nursing mothers, it can improve the milk flow, especially in conjunction with alfalfa sprouts. Anaemia is a common sign of deficiency, along with muscle weakness, lack of energy, loss of appetite, digestive disturbances, abdominal distension, diarrhoea, sleeplessness, forgetfulness and irritability.

Hint: Make sure you are getting adequate food sources of folic acid such as: brewer's yeast, torula yeast, black-eyed beans, wheatgerm, bran, all legumes, green vegetables and nuts. Liver is the only significant meat source, although it is quite unnecessary to partake of second-hand folic acid when so much is available from natural sources.

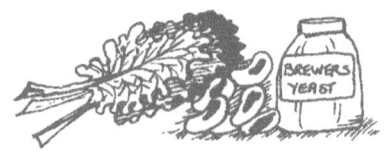

Inositol

Inositol is still part of the B-complex group and, with choline, part of lecithin. Think of inositol, choline and biotin as fat metabolisers and contributors as far as avoiding cholesterol build-up. As a component of lecithin, it mixes in most liquids, particularly in fruit juices. Lecithin is also an excellent way to maximise the effectiveness of vitamin E.

Heat and light destroy inositol, and coffee and lindane are two additional disruptive factors. Lindane is a chemical pesticide of the chlorinated hydrocarbon family which includes DDT.

Eczema and sometimes digestive problems, especially with fats, are definite deficiency symptoms. Premature hair loss is also a key indicator that the diet is deficient in inositol and should be treated immediately by supplementary lecithin.

The scalp reacts to a deficiency of choline by loss of hair colour, to a deficiency of biotin by the appearance of dandruff, and to a deficiency of inositol with hair loss. This proves how closely these three vitamins work together. If your hair is receding or you are showing any other of the symptoms mentioned you should study these vitamins and their relationship to inositol in maintaining the body's optimum health.

Inositol is found in the same foods and similar concentrations as choline, but now some fruits are being included in the list of abundant sources such as: oranges, grapefruit, raisins, cantaloupes and peaches.

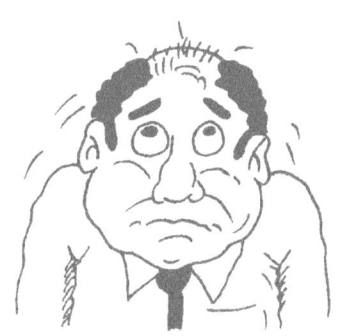

Paba (Para-Aminobenzoic Acid)

One of the newest members of the B-complex group and also water-soluble, PABA can be synthesised in the body. However, therapeutic dosages are necessary for it to have its most beneficial effects.

Deficiency symptoms are similar to those of inositol. It has been known to aid in the natural recolouring of faded hair in conjunction with choline and B5. Some of you may know of its effectiveness as a sunscreen and how it forms an essential ingredient in every effective suntan lotion or cream.

In general terms, foods found to be abundant sources of other B vitamins are certain to be valuable sources of PABA.

Vitamin C – Ascorbic Acid

Most animals synthesise their own vitamin C, but humans, apes and guinea pigs must rely upon dietary sources. Water-soluble vitamin C plays a primary role in the formation of collagen, which is important for the growth and repair of body tissue cells, gums, blood vessels, bones and teeth. It also helps in the body's absorption of iron.

Probably the greatest depletion of the body's absorption and utilisation of vitamin C is caused by stress, not to mention smoking cigarettes or even worse drugs. Cooking in copper pots along with modern food processing and refining robs us of vital vitamin C even before food gets to the table. Surely it must be a great revelation to you all that raw foods can give us a fighting chance to build strong bodies free of disease and great minds capable of learning so much more than we give ourselves credit for.

A deficiency of vitamin C can be a cause of cancer in many of the body's organs. Captain Cook created history by becoming one of the first sailors to prevent death from scurvy among his crew, simply by feeding them fresh limes. In many ways, this was more significant than finding new land for the British Crown.

Vitamin C is vital for the maintenance and health of collagen in every body cell. It helps to heal wounds and burns, broken bones and bleeding gums, and aids in the maintenance of the white blood corpuscles (which surround damaged or infected tissue to isolate the condition) and of the adrenal glands (which aid the balancing of our emotions). In combination with vitamin E it works to strengthen the infant after childbirth if mother's health is below par.

Further benefits of vitamin C are the detoxification of poisons and the lowering of blood clot incidence in the veins and varicose veins. There is so much more that can be said about vitamin C and all the wonderful things it can do for you. If you include the following foods in your diet you will never have to worry about getting enough of this vitamin.

The richest sources are: guavas, blackcurrants, Brussels sprouts, parsley, capsicum, broccoli, watercress, pawpaw, red cabbage and kohlrabi, all of which possess above 60mg per 100g edible portion. Other fruits and vegetables, freshly sprouted legumes and seeds are also very rich sources of vitamin C.

Vitamin D – The Sunshine Vitamin

Vitamin D can be stored in the body for quite some time. Sunshine and natural foods are vital ingredients to human health, but when out of proportion to human needs, a disease such as rickets will manifest. Thanks to the recognition of the essential nutritional role of vitamin D, rickets is a disease rarely encountered in the Western world today. An adult form of rickets, osteomalacia, is not a common problem, however the symptoms include a compressed ribcage, wrists and ankles appearing swollen, arms and legs becoming bowed, excessive perspiration during sleep and distension of the abdomen. Continuous bowel trouble and spinal curvature are also obvious signs and this occurs more with older people. Other less frequent symptoms are severe tooth decay and osteoporosis (bone calcium deficiency caused by inadequate utilisation of calcium from the diet due to a lack of vitamin D).

This vitamin is vital for the utilisation of calcium and phosphorus and is used in the treatment of conjunctivitis, also aiding the body in the assimilation of vitamin A.

Food sources are: butter, sunflower seed kernels, liver, eggs, mushrooms, natural cheeses and seafoods. The sun's rays are a vital source. Another source is milk, however this is a poor source for humans.

Vitamin E – Alpha Tocopherol

Alpha is one of the eight chemicals classified in the tocopherols group. There are two forms of tocopherol available for therapeutic application. D-alpha tocopherol acetate is known as 'natural' – derived from natural sources – and Dl-alpha tocopherol acetate is regarded as 'synthetic' and not as potent.

Vitamin E is insoluble in water and soluble in fat. It is stored in the liver, fatty tissues, heart, muscles, blood and many of the body's glands, but for a short time only.

If fats in the gastrointestinal tract are in any way spoilt or rancid, vitamin E absorption will be severely limited. One of the important functions of vitamin E is to prevent fats becoming rancid and this can only occur if the vitamin E is assimilable. Then it can do its work in protecting vitamins A and C from oxidation loss and the unsaturated oils from rancidity. Heat and oxygen are two of the major causes of rancidity and loss of vitamin E. Chlorine in drinking water is also a loss-causing influence, again emphasising the importance of a water purifier ensuring the consumption of distilled or filtered water. Long storage in freezers and modern processing techniques also cause a loss of vitamin E.

Women experience losses caused by oral contraceptives or any other hormone intake, and by the changes taking place in their body while going through menopause, or when pregnant or nursing. The human heart works so hard from birth until death. It is often abused by unsuitable nutrition and unbalanced emotions. Quite often, if the nutritional aspect is attended to first, then emotional problems are overcome later.

This vitamin minimises the effects of pollution and passive smoking. Other benefits of vitamin E include its ability to help arteries expand, thereby stimulating circulation to avert strokes, carrying the improved blood circulation right to the surface of the skin where its healing will become speedier. It will help overcome varicose veins, cystic mastitis and will even delay ageing. Vitamin E aids the reproductive systems of both males and females by improving virility and the condition of the sperm, as well as strengthening the female abdominal membranes to avert a spontaneous abortion or miscarriage.

Skin problems ranging from ulcers, open sores, severe burns and gangrene have been known to respond significantly to vitamin E as the major form of treatment.

Best food sources are: wheatgerm oil, sunflower seeds, sunflower oil, safflower oil, almonds, other vegetable oils, wheatgerm and peanuts.

Vitamin K – Phytonadione

Vitamin K is a fat-soluble vitamin essential in the formation of prothrombin, a blood-clotting chemical. Haemophilia (excessive bleeding due to inefficient blood clotting, often inherited, but sometimes found to be congenital) is occasionally a nutritional-deficiency condition in which vitamin D plays a leading role. Colitis, related to inadequate bowel bacteria and resulting in smelly stools, can also indicate lack of adequate vitamin K in the body (as well as incorrect food or indigestion). Coeliac disease (gluten intolerance) also responds to increased vitamin K by consuming far more green vegetables, especially alfalfa.

It is quite incredible when you think about it that we do not bleed to death when we experience a tiny cut to our skin. This is due to vitamin K ensuring the formation of the blood-clotting chemical, prothrombin. Vitamin K also prevents internal haemorrhaging, aids in the regulation of menstrual flow and helps sufferers from irregular nose bleeding.

Best food sources are: all green vegetables, alfalfa sprouts, liver, cheese, butter, whole grains, yoghurt, vegetable oils and, to a lesser degree, egg yolk.

Vitamin P – Bioflavonoids

The bioflavonoids are necessary to the proper functioning and absorption of vitamin C. The group of compounds comprises rutin, hesperidin, flavones and flavals. The flavonoids are the compounds found in the pith of citrus fruits and their role in maintaining capillary permeability gives this group the name of vitamin P.

If you bruise easily, or your gums bleed frequently, especially after cleaning teeth, and you are susceptible to many infectious conditions, chances are you are deficient in the bioflavonoids.

Vitamin P works to maintain a more robust skin and a greater effectiveness of vitamins C and E, helping women especially with menopause, particularly in regard to the balancing of physical and emotional discomforts.

By far the best natural food source of vitamin P is the white pith under the skin of citrus fruits. For this important reason, only the outer, coloured skin should be removed, leaving plenty of pith around the inside flesh.

MINERALS

A total of 103 elements have been discovered so far to be part of nature on Earth. The four main elements are: oxygen, carbon, hydrogen and nitrogen. These four main elements make up around 96% of the human body. The remaining 4% is composed of mineral elements.

Minerals are as important to the human body as a set of spark plugs is for a car. When even one mineral is lacking from the diet, the result is felt by the entire body and the role of certain vitamins will also be inhibited, which leads to even more problems such as general ill health, lack of energy, feeling of irritability, nervous disorders, and muscular and mental deterioration.

As minerals are part of every living cell in the body, they are closely integrated with one another and perform a multitude of functions. With a raw food diet you can be sure of getting the minerals in a balanced form.

Calcium – Ca

Alkaline mineral

The human body is composed of more calcium than any other mineral. About 90% is contained in the bone structure, the frame of the body.

Calcium is important to nerve, muscle and metabolic functions, as well as blood coagulation. Its absorption is inhibited by oxalic acid (from coffee, tea, cocoa, meat and rhubarb) and sucrose. Vitamin D helps absorption.

Cancer research has shown that cancerous tissues are abnormally low in calcium. Due to lack of calcium, these cancer cells will spread to other parts of the body. Excess intake of fatty-based foods hinders calcium absorption. Most people think that they will only get calcium from dairy and associated products. Nothing could be further from the truth.

The following foods will give you adequate calcium: sesame seeds, kelp, collard and kale leaves, turnip greens, soya beans, most nuts, parsley, dandelion greens, watercress, chickpeas, white beans, pinto beans, figs, sunflower seeds, beetroot greens, wheat bran, mung beans, olives, broccoli, broad beans, spinach, prunes, lentils, rice bran, cowpeas, lima beans, chives, peanuts, lettuce, apricots, savoy cabbage, raisins, blackcurrants, dates, snap beans, leeks, pumpkin seeds, green onions, parsnip, oranges, celery, cashew nuts, rye grain, carrots and many other foods in lesser amounts. Do yourself a favour and seek your calcium requirements in natural foods before looking to the cow!

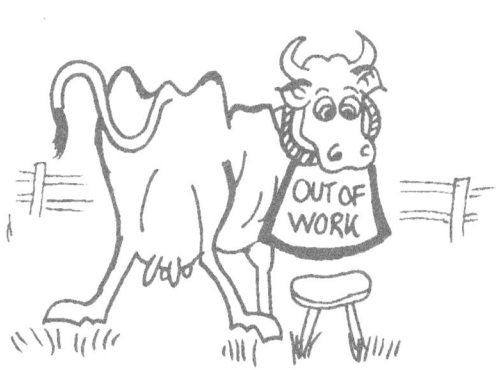

Chlorine – Cl

Acid mineral

Organic chlorine is essential for the production of vital gastric juices, which aid digestion. Chlorine foods stimulate hydrochloric acid (HCL) production and help to eliminate poisons from the body and assist in purifying the blood.

Weight watchers will be happy to know that an increase in chlorine-rich foods will help you to stay slim as they cleanse the body of excess fats. High intakes of chlorine, however, can create toxicity, as can sodium, so care should be taken to avoid common salt wherever possible – over 15g daily is regarded as high and is easily achieved since chlorine is also present in our water supplies.

Natural sources are: tomato, celery, lettuce, cabbage, spinach, parsnip, rhubarb, eggplant, cucumber, avocado, sweet potato, dates, dandelion greens, cauliflower, carrots, leek, raspberry, beetroot, banana, pineapple, limes, chives, raisins, mango, artichoke, blackberry, guava, potato, lentils, peas, onion, strawberry, watermelon, sweet corn, figs, chick peas, sunflower seeds, brazil nuts, peaches, beans, cherry, hazelnuts, soya beans and grapes.

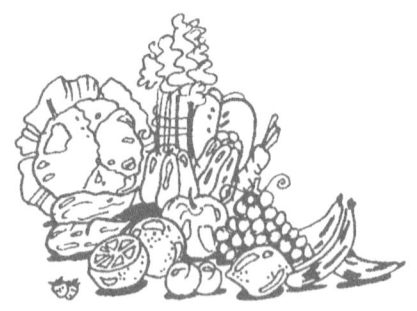

Copper – Cu

Acid mineral

Copper is rarely deficient in the body. When deficiency occurs, it is usually found in third world people.

Most of the copper content of the body is stored in the muscles, liver and bones. Copper is a trace mineral and part of every body tissue. Copper helps with proper assimilation of iron and improves the functions of the digestive system. Foods rich in copper assist tissue respiration and protect the lungs from infection.

Copper is required by the body to convert iron into blood haemoglobin, for oxidising ascorbic acid and converting it to vitamin C, and for oxidising the protein tyrosine, by which its work on the pigmentation of skin and hair is accomplished.

Most suitable sources of copper are: nuts, legumes, grains and prunes.

Fluorine – F

Acid mineral

Fluorine is an excellent beauty mineral and found throughout the human body. It helps to preserve youth and gives a sparkle to your eyes, maintaining delicate functions of the iris in the eye. In its natural form as calcium fluoride (available from nuts and green vegetables), it strengthens bones, teeth, nails and eyes. However, the quantity found in modern man is close to toxic level, because so many city water authorities have included sodium fluoride in our water. If fluoridated water is taken excessively, it has a toxic effect on the body which can reduce the body's ability to absorb calcium and therefore have subsequent deficiency effects. A fluorine deficiency may lead to retarded growth, a decalcifying effect on the bones, and impaired kidney, liver, heart and nervous and glandular systems.

Foods high in fluorine are: asparagus, oats, garlic, rice, cabbage, goats milk, watercress, rice bran, beetroot, endive, corn, barley, millet, wheat, fresh vegetables and fresh fruits

Iodine – I

Acid mineral

Iodine is essential for regulating the thyroid gland. Iodine is stored in the thyroid gland and its purpose is to control the metabolism of the entire body. Iodine foods assist in regulating the body's metabolism and activity, thereby affecting growth, development and the rate of digestion. Iodine foods assist the body to burn up excess fat. Goitre, which is a thyroid enlargement and leads to a slow rate of hormone secretion, is a deficiency of iodine.

Irregular heartbeat, hardening of the arteries, rapid pulse, nervousness, irritability, dry hair, obesity and poor mental abilities, such as lack of concentration, are all attributable to lack of iodine.

Food sources are: seafood, kelp, pineapple, eggs, cheddar cheese, onions and vegetables grown in iodine-rich soils. Kelp is an excellent source of iodine for vegetarians.

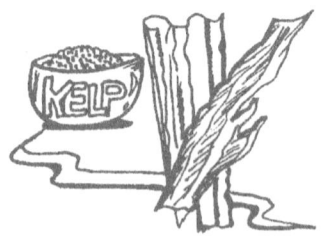

Iron – Fe

Alkaline mineral

Iron is the nucleus of every cell in the body. It is essential in the formation of rich red blood cells. 90% of iron is contained in the blood. A combination of protein and iron is required for the formation of blood haemoglobin. Iron foods improve protein metabolism.

If you are suffering from dizziness, anaemia, fevers, muscle fatigue, mental fatigue, and have difficulty breathing, are faint or experience constipation this could be a sign that you need to increase iron-rich foods. Continual drinking of coffee and tea retard the absorption of this mineral, which is so important for the formation of myoglobin that is essential for oxygen distribution to all the body's muscular cells. If you take laxatives you also delay the absorption of iron.

Best food sources are: yeasts, rice bran, liver (but remember this contains much of the animal's toxicity so is not recommended), wheat bran, pumpkin seeds, beans, seeds, nuts, eggs and parsley (a must in every salad). Iron is also found in smaller amounts in: dulse, kelp, sesame seeds, soya beans, most sprouted beans, beetroot greens, dandelion, spinach, dates, figs, fennel, barley, kale leaves, lettuce, peas and turnips.

Magnesium – Mg

Alkaline mineral

Magnesium is essential for the formation of strong bones and teeth. It is necessary for calcium metabolism and vital for efficient nerve and muscle functioning, as well as for converting blood sugar into energy. A deficiency leads to hardening of the arteries and high blood pressure. Alcohol consumption leads to a magnesium deficiency and causes a deficiency in most other minerals.

Major food sources are: wheat bran and germ, nuts, buckwheat, dietary yeasts, beans, grains, dried fruits and vegetables, especially the greens.

Manganese – Ma

Alkaline mineral

Manganese is important in bile production and in some hormone and enzyme functions. The majority of manganese in the body is found in the liver, pancreas and the adrenal glands. This mineral is essential for regulating menstrual periods, for expectant mothers and during lactation. Manganese is a good memory builder, essential for effective protein, fat and carbohydrate metabolism, and as a source of energy. Manganese foods assist in hormone production. Both males and females need manganese foods for healthy sex hormone production.

Best food sources are: most nuts including coconut, buckwheat, barley, kidney beans, Lima beans, pineapple, grapes, beetroot, parsley, lettuce, watercress, apricots, bananas, cherries, green beans, kale, artichoke, avocado, blackberries, dates, carrots, celery, cucumber, dandelion, figs, lemons, pears, apples, melons, parsnips and chives.

Phosphorus – P

Acid mineral

The maintenance and repair of the entire nervous system depends on phosphorus. Phosphorus is important in assisting vital energy distribution throughout the entire body, keeps acids out of the bloodstream and assists the transportation of fatty acids around the body.

A lack of phosphorus may lead to poor memory and weak abilities of concentration. Phosphorus foods strengthen the nervous system and are essential for the health of the skin, hair, nails and brain. They also improve blood circulation and normalise blood pressure levels especially for those people who have a very low blood pressure count.

Sources of phosphorus are: all calcium-rich foods with the addition of wild rice, barley, sorghum, kelp, garlic, mushrooms and peas.

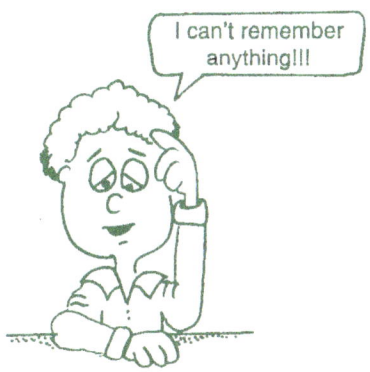

Potassium – K

Alkaline mineral

Its primary role in health is working within the body's cells to regulate water balance, normalise heart rhythms and strengthen the heart muscles. Cancer cells cannot live in a solution of potassium. This mineral assists in the elimination of blood impurities via the kidneys, prevents hardening of the arteries, balances acid and alkaline levels in the body, assists with repair of the liver and is essential for the formation of glycogen from the liver. This substance is stored and converted in the liver to glucose, which is a useable energy source. Potassium is the most effective healing mineral for the body. Cooking and processing easily destroy the potassium content of foods.

Deficiency symptoms are irritability, weariness, sleepwalking and poor nerves. Diabetics are often potassium deficient.

Foods rich in potassium are: dietary yeasts, soya beans and soya products, other beans, dried fruits, bran, sunflower seed kernels, parsley, nuts and fresh green olives. Containing lesser amounts are: bananas, carrots, celery, pumpkin, beetroot, radish, peas and barley.

Silicon – Si

Acid mineral

Silicon is one of the most abundant minerals in the soil. In fresh fruits and vegetables, silicon is mainly concentrated in the outer skin layer. These foods are essential for healthy hair, skin and teeth, and keeping you looking beautiful! Silicon is also a cleansing mineral, a protector against mental fatigue, nervous exhaustion, baldness, infection and poor vision. The action of silicon is dependent on the mineral fluorine.

A deficiency is often related to the formation of arthritic conditions.

Best food sources are: lettuce (a few leaves for minimum daily needs), parsnip, asparagus, rice bran and all fruits and vegetables. Avocado, walnuts, peanuts and almonds are also good sources of silicon and have been used as natural ingredients in special skin creams.

Sodium – Na

Alkaline mineral

Sodium works with other minerals in the blood to maintain their solubility, but high intakes of it can be dangerous to the health, especially from common salt, which contributes to cardiovascular problems from cramps to heart attacks. There is no need to add salt to our food. To me, it would be an insult if someone proceeded to put salt on food I served them, especially before they even tasted it! Natural food has the correct balance of the mineral sodium.

Best food sources are: eggs, meat, celery, most chlorine foods as listed above with the addition of cashews, rice, wheat bran, kumquat, wild rice, pear, nectarine, broccoli, Brussels sprouts, endive and olives.

Sulphur – S

Acid mineral

Sulphur is essential for maintaining correct brain functioning through the regulation of the body's oxygen balance, for balanced functioning of liver and bile secretion, and for maintaining healthy skin, hair and nails.

Take care when eating sulphur-dried fruits (the bright-coloured apricots, peaches and nectarines) for the sulphurous acid will impair the kidneys. Sulphur-rich foods assist growth in children and prevent the development of infections such as hepatitis.

Remember, cooking destroys the sulphur content of foods.

Food sources are: Brazil and most other nuts, meat and fish, eggs, watercress, beans and green leafy vegetables. Avocado, tomato, sweet corn, onion, mushrooms, barley, rhubarb, watermelon, strawberry, apple, oranges and limes are also good sources.

Zinc – Zn

Acid mineral

If you are constantly tired, not alert, have poor hair condition, susceptible to colds and lack sex drive, consider this mineral.

Regular consumption of alcohol can lead to a zinc deficiency. Zinc is vital for the body's enzyme systems and every man and woman should be sure to consume adequate amounts of zinc through their food.

Wonderful food sources available are: pumpkin seeds, nuts, egg yolk, rye, wheatgerm and brewer's yeast.

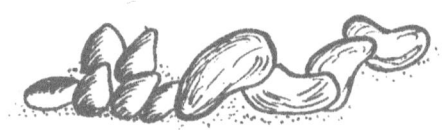

TRACE MINERALS

Aluminium – Al

Trace mineral

There is no recognised need for aluminium to be part of human nutrition. Excess consumption of aluminium can be fatal. The average daily amount ingested from the diet has been estimated to range from 10mg to 100mg.

Cooking with aluminium cookware, cutlery and use of aluminium food wraps are the main sources of this trace mineral. Excess aluminium in the blood will lead to poisoning.

Cobalt – Co

Trace mineral

Its presence is vital to the red blood cells. It is part of the B12 structure. Cobalt must be supplied from the diet. It cannot be synthesised by the body.

Such foods as fish and all seafoods are reliable sources of cobalt, but do not overlook traces that are present in most foods, especially whole grains, alfalfa and other green vegetables.

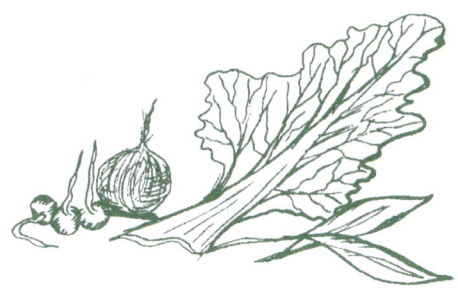

Mercury – Hg

Trace mineral

Mercury is not an essential trace mineral. Mercury is widely distributed in the outer atmosphere and is also part of some chemical fertilisers, pesticides and other by-products from some factories. Mercury is a threat to the environment and the human body.

Fish from inland waters are often contaminated with mercury, as a result of factories that dump waste products into the rivers and sea. Excess mercury will have adverse effects on the functioning of the entire nervous system.

Molybdenum – Mo

Trace mineral

Molybdenum is part of two essential enzymes – xanthine and aldehyde oxidase. Xanthine is required for the oxidation of fats. The nervous system and brain also require molybdenum. It is obtainable from both plant and animal sources.

Legumes and green leafy vegetables are a very good source of this essential trace mineral (depending on the soil condition).

Selenium – Se

Trace mineral

An essential trace mineral, selenium functions are closely related to vitamin E. With antioxidant properties that help the body to utilise oxygen, Selenium also delays the rate of oxidation of polyunsaturated fatty acids, which is vital for the preservation and elasticity of all skin tissues. The selenium content of food is directly related to the condition of the soil. A selenium deficiency is related to premature ageing and selenium has also been successfully used in the treatment of Kwashiorkor (a protein deficiency disease).

Best food sources are: whole grains, wheatgerm, Brazil nuts, alfalfa sprouts, mushrooms and most other vegetables, with traces in most fruits. Other sources are: organ meat, seafood, other meat and garlic, but sufficient will be available from the natural foods diet.

OTHER MINERALS

There are many more minerals not listed that are gaining recognition as vital to human needs, guaranteeing them inclusion in the expanding list of essential trace minerals. These now include: rubidium, strontium, boron, bromine, barium, chromium, arsenic and vanadium. Other trace minerals known to reside within the human body, which are primarily 'non-essential' are: zirconium, lead, niobium, cadmium, tellurium, titanium, tin, nickel, gold, lithium, antimony, bismuth, silver, caesium, uranium, beryllium, radium and probably many more that are so far too rare to have been recognised. And when they are recognised, no doubt there will be many evils and perhaps benefits associated with them that we will learn to understand.

When I think about the vulnerability of minerals and their relationship to our wellbeing, I realise that the elements are really stacked against us until we learn to eat our foods naturally. All the processing and extra fuss that goes along with preparation of our food is not only robbing us of vital minerals but of the chance for our bodies to function as they truly should. Learn about minerals and respect them by not murdering your vegetables and you will discover the real body you were meant to have.

Anne Clark

The previous information on vitamins is a basic guide, which I would encourage you to explore further.

Recommended books for further reading are:

- *New Dimensions in Health: From soil to psyche* by David A. Phillips

- *Reader's Digest Family Guide to Alternative Medicine*

- *Fit for Life* by Harvey and Marilyn Diamond

- *Nutrients to Age without Senility* by Dr Abram Hoffer

- *Laugh with Health: Your complete guide to health, diet, nutrition and natural foods* by Manfred Urs Koch.

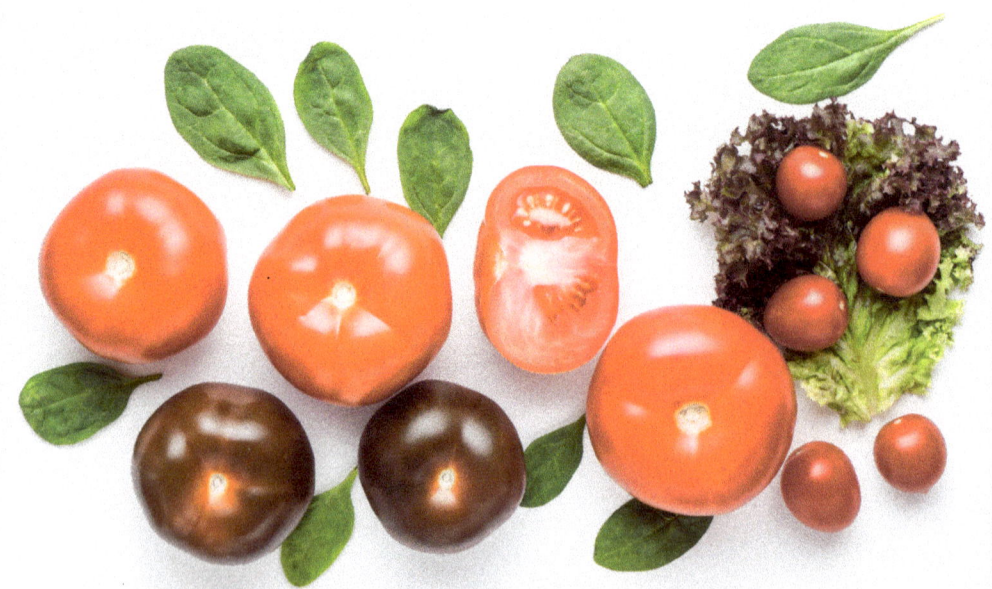

 # Digestion – what's it all about

Few of us really understand the digestive system as well as we should. The most familiar aspects of food processing, eating and defecation are automatically controlled. After its entrance through the mouth, the food we eat takes a long and eventful journey through the digestive tract before part of it is eliminated through the anus.

If we understand just enough about digestion to realise what happens to our food once we have finished chewing and enjoying various tastes then this will help us to further respect just what we do put in our mouths and, in particular, the way we combine one food with another. The digestive tract, also called the alimentary canal, is a tube about 4.4m (15ft) long, extending from the mouth, where food is taken in, to the anus, the exit for elimination of unused food. Below the diaphragm, the digestive tract is referred to as the gastrointestinal tract. The digestive tube is like a long, coiled hose of varying diameter. Each section of it has a slightly different structure and function, and each may be considered an organ in its own right.

Special organs that produce digestive juices are situated along the length of the digestive system. These organs include the salivary glands, stomach, liver, pancreas, gall bladder and the small intestine.

The overall functions of the digestive system are to receive food, grind it into small particles and chemically change the food into a form that can be absorbed and used by the body. Some food material, such as the fibre in fruits and vegetables, cannot be chemically broken down and so leaves the body through the anus as waste material or faeces. The salivary glands, liver and pancreas release chemicals that are necessary to change food into the simple forms which can be easily absorbed by our body.

The tongue is an important part of the digestive system. Four flavours are identified by sense organs in the tongue. According to Ayurvedic principles the taste buds on our tongue are organised in six groups: sweet, sour, salty, bitter, pungent and astringent. These six basic tastes are derived from a mixture of the five elements: Earth, Water, Fire, Air and Space. The digestive system responds via the sense organs of the tongue.

To understand the functions of the stomach and intestines properly, we must understand about the food we eat.

Carbohydrates are chemical compounds made up of carbon, hydrogen and oxygen. Most of the carbohydrates we eat are used by the body to generate energy.

Rice, bread, potatoes, honey, corn, millet, cereals, fruits are examples of carbohydrates.

Fats and oils are also compounds of carbon, hydrogen and oxygen. They are also used to produce energy for the body. Excess fats and oils are stored as a fatty layer under the skin or around organs. The main difference between fats and oils is that fats are solid at room temperature, whereas oils are liquids.

Fats are found in seeds, butter, milk, cheese and meat. Oils are found in corn, peanuts, castor-oil seeds and coconuts.

Proteins are very complicated compounds made up of units called amino acids. They are used to build tissues for growth and repair.

Proteins are found in vegetables and fruits, nuts and seeds, meat, eggs, milk, cheese and fish.

The food we eat is first chewed into small pieces. Often it is not chewed long enough and this creates more problems and more work for the rest of the digestion. Saliva, which contains a special digestive substance, begins the first stage of digestion. It also acts as a lubricant and makes food easier to swallow. Food continues on into the stomach, where digestion continues with the help of more digestive juices, and then into the small intestine where digestion is completed. The digested food is then absorbed through the walls of the small intestine into the blood. The small intestine is about seven metres long.

THE PROCESSES OF DIGESTION

The digestion of food involves two processes:

1. **Mechanical digestion, which** consists of various movements that aid chemical digestion. The teeth first break up food before it is swallowed. Then the muscles of the stomach and small intestine churn the food so that it is thoroughly mixed with the digestive juices.

2. **Chemical digestion, which** is the process in which the large molecules of carbohydrates, fats and oils, and proteins are broken down into molecules small enough to pass through the

walls of the small intestine into the blood. This chemical process needs the presence of special substances called enzymes which are found in digestive juices.

The teeth and the tongue aid in mechanical digestion. The teeth break up the food so that it can mix more easily with the saliva, which is a digestive juice produced by salivary glands. There are three pairs of salivary glands, which produce more than one litre of saliva per day. The saliva contains an enzyme (salivary amylase) which can change starch into the double sugar, maltose.

The tongue helps mix the food and then rolls it into a ball for swallowing. Digestion by saliva continues in the stomach for about 20 minutes until the action of the enzyme is stopped by the gastric juices of the stomach. However, carbohydrate digestion continues in the small intestine with the conversion of the molecules of maltose and other sugars to simpler molecules which can be absorbed. Maltose, lactose (milk sugar) and sucrose (cane sugar) need the action of enzymes to change them to the simple sugars glucose, fructose and galactose.

The pancreas releases an enzyme into the duodenum to convert any unchanged starch to maltose. This enzyme, found in the pancreatic juice, is called pancreatic amylase. In the ileum, maltose, sucrose, and lactose are changed by other enzymes into simple sugars. Carbohydrate digestion is now complete, and the simple sugars pass into the bloodstream. Cellulose, a carbohydrate found in fresh fruit and vegetables, cannot be digested by the human body, but plays an important part because it helps the movement of food substances through the digestive system.

In the Raw

The stomach lies in the upper part of the abdomen, just below the diaphragm. Food is brought to the stomach from the mouth through a tube, the oesophagus, which passes through the diaphragm. Consider the stomach as the passageway for food extending from the mouth to the anus. The stomach has many functions which include storage of food which has been chewed by the teeth and then swallowed, mixing of the food with digestive juices, controlling the release of food into the small intestine, killing bacteria present in the food and generally giving you a hard time if you don't combine your food correctly. While food is in the stomach, it is churned and thoroughly mixed by the movements of the stomach wall, it becomes a semi-liquid form called chyme. When it is filled the stomach may hold up to 1.5 litres of food and liquid. The stomach empties all its contents into the duodenum two to six hours after a meal is eaten. Food, which is made up mainly of carbohydrates, leaves the stomach after two or three hours. Protein-rich foods are slower in leaving the

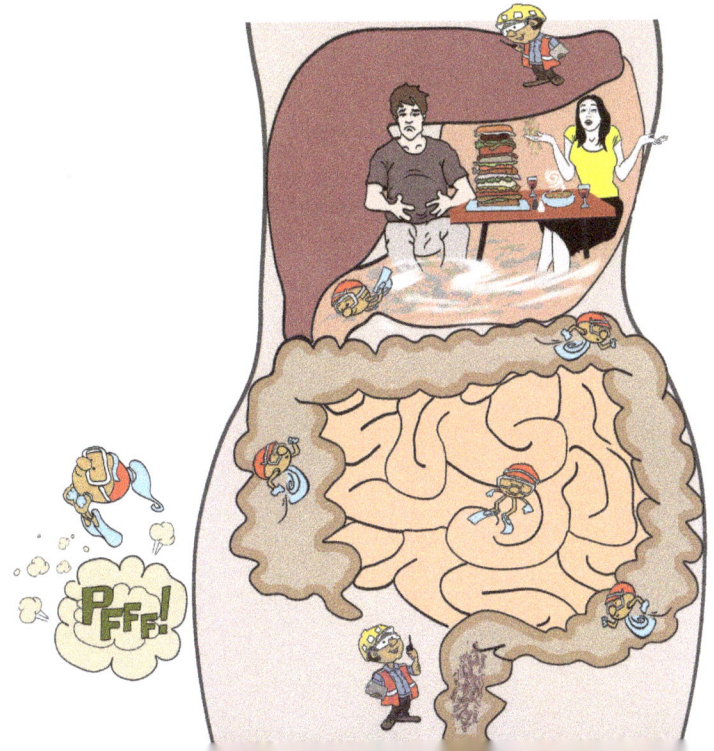

stomach and foods high in fats may take up to six hours to leave the stomach. If food is taken into the stomach before adequate breakdown of the previous meal's proteins, the pylorus (the lower escape valve) may be forced to allow the premature evacuation of some or all of the inadequately prepared food, placing a real burden on the facilities of the lower gastrointestinal tract.

Mechanical digestion continues in the stomach as the food is churned by muscular contraction of the stomach walls. Gastric juice contains hydrochloric acid and digestive enzymes. It also contains mucus, a sticky substance that forms a protective coating on the stomach wall. In adults, proteins are broken up by an enzyme called pepsin. This is easy to remember really, I just think of P for protein and P for pepsin. Pepsin works efficiently in the acidic environment of the stomach but becomes inactive in the alkaline environment of the intestine. If a protein food is accompanied by starch-concentrated food (i.e. eating meat with potatoes/bread or sweets), fermentation will usually result.

You are probably wondering why the enzyme pepsin does not digest the protein in the stomach cells at the same time as it digests the protein in food. In other words, why doesn't the stomach digest itself? It is because, firstly, pepsin is produced in an inactive form called pepsinogen, which only becomes active when it mixes with the hydrochloric acid in the stomach. Secondly, the stomach lining is protected by a thick coating of mucus. It is important to note that all highly seasoned and spiced foods should be avoided indefinitely if you suffer peptic and duodenal ulcers, for strong curries, peppers and spices are known to be responsible for inducing damage to the sensitive linings of the gastrointestinal tract.

An infant's stomach produces an enzyme called rennin, which is important in the digestion of mother's milk. Rennin begins to diminish when the teeth begin to form. Nature has it all worked out! By the time the child has a full set of first teeth and is able to thoroughly chew solid foods, the gastric juice no longer contains rennin. Without this enzyme milk is no longer an acceptable food in its liquid state. Its continued consumption is considered by some to result in probable indigestion and possible allergies. It is beyond me why so many people still consume cow's milk. Milk creates several problems in the stomach. The alkaline nature of milk reduces the effectiveness of hydrochloric acid digestion and, if the milk is taken in with other animal protein, large quantities of mucus are secreted as the stomach attempts to compensate for the lack of rennin. This secretion is delayed for a time by the fat coating the gastric mucosa. Eventually it will make its way through, but the milk will have become soured in the heat of the stomach and that is just another bad ending!

When the food leaves the stomach, it enters the first part of the small intestine, the duodenum. Don't ask me who dreamed up all these names of our various body parts; I guess they wanted to really make people work when it comes to learning about the human body. The duodenum is about 25cm long and leads into a much longer section, the jejunum, which is about 210cm in length. The remainder of the small intestine is called the ileum, which is about 450cm long. The total length of the small intestine is therefore about seven metres.

Food is moved through the small intestine by means of a process called peristalsis. Digestion, which began in the mouth and stomach, is completed in the small intestine. Enzymes are released from the pancreas and special cells in the lining of the intestine. Bile is secreted from the liver to help the digestion of fats and oils. Imagine the inner wall of the small intestine, with its velvety appearance due to the presence of many tiny finger-like projections called villi. These villi greatly increase the rate at which digested food can be absorbed. Ultimately, food ends up in your blood. It passes through the walls of the villi into the blood vessels inside each villus. The blood carrying the dissolved food materials is then carried by the hepatic portal vein to the liver. The liver either stores the excess food materials or releases them as required. However, the products of protein digestion are not stored.

Undigested food (mainly cellulose fibres from fruits and vegetables) leaves the small intestine and passes into the large intestine known as the colon. Within the colon, water, mineral salts, water-soluble vitamins and sometimes toxic bacteria are absorbed into the blood. The toxic bacteria are another story, however, if you eat natural foods, exercise, rest and play, you may never have to worry about it. If you abuse your body you pay the price! The final residue, the faeces, collects in the rectum from where it is eliminated.

Some of you may be familiar with carbohydrate loading, where you eat a lot of carbohydrates; and excess glucose resulting from digestion is stored in the liver as glycogen or changed into fat. When the body needs more energy, such as when we are exercising, the stored glycogen can be readily converted into glucose. In times of starvation, the fat deposits in our body can be broken down to glucose to release energy. Carbohydrate loading is not necessarily healthy. I believe that any time the body is overfed we are putting great strain on our digestion and liver and winning the race means nothing to me if my health is at risk.

If we eat too much protein, the excess amino acids resulting from digestion cannot be stored. The protein must be treated in some way. First, the amino acid molecules are broken down into two parts. One part, which contains the element nitrogen, is converted in the liver into a harmless nitrogen compound called urea, which is excreted by the kidneys. The second part is changed into glucose, which may be stored or used immediately. Too much protein makes too much work for your body, and the result is disease and a body that does not function as it should.

For years, nutritionists and doctors alike have been telling us to eat plenty of protein and stressing it should be animal protein. Let's look at this from another point of view. If you had one acre of average quality land and wanted to get the maximum amount of protein that you could use for human consumption out of it, what would you choose to do with it?

Would you believe me if I told you soya beans work out to be 20 times more efficient than growing meat? Furthermore, vegetable sources of protein will give you many times more protein than even the best animal source (milk). So you'd be silly to use your precious land for beef, wouldn't you? Unless you were being coerced by economic pressure to produce beef. We can influence the way our world goes about producing its food. The average meat-eating Westerner eats their way through 1,000 kilograms of grain every year. 93% of this is eaten indirectly in the form of meat and meat products.

If the Western world was to cut its meat consumption by just 50%, each person doing so would release enough grain to keep two more people alive who may otherwise starve. 95% of the soya bean harvest, which is one of the greatest sources of protein in the world, is fed straight to animals. Only 1.5% of the crop is used directly by humans. What is going on in this world? Why have we gone so far off the track?

Finally, plant protein molecules are simpler and smaller than those of flesh proteins. They are thus easier to digest and have no inherent toxic wastes. Humans have the choice of consuming first-hand proteins, produced by nature, or second-hand proteins, from animal flesh. Perhaps you will consider a vegetarian diet now that you know how sensitive the human digestive system is and how sensitive and vulnerable the world is becoming. You will see that you can make a difference to both the environment and yourself by what you eat.

HEALTH ISSUES FROM POOR DIGESTION

Stomach ulcers

In a normal functioning digestive system, the stomach wall is protected from attack by acids and enzymes by its thick surface layer of mucus. The protection fails to work when people continue to eat poorly, suffer emotional stress and hold in their emotions over a long period of time. Part of the stomach lining is therefore attacked by gastric juices forming an ulcer or sore spot. If the damage continues, blood vessels may be broken and bleeding commences. In extreme cases, a hole may develop right through the stomach wall, and food may escape, causing serious infection. This type of ulcer is called a perforated ulcer. Ulcers may form in the first part of the duodenum if excessive gastric juice pours out into the duodenum from the stomach. These are called duodenal ulcers.

Indigestion

What is indigestion anyway? I've always felt it is a feeling of discomfort in the stomach. Some people call it 'heartburn' – a strange term, as if your heart was burning (on fire) you would be dead or close to it! Sometimes a person feels uncomfortable because there is air in the stomach. Indigestion may be caused by eating unusual food, i.e. food which is cooked (this is unusual for me), food which is not part of the usual diet, too much food (usually the problem) or nervous tension (nearly always the problem). In short, indigestion is a sign from your body to your brain that you are doing something wrong. Listen to your body while you still have a brain!

Constipation and diarrhoea

Two of my favourite subjects! Not really!

Constipation is a condition in which the rectum or bowel is not emptied often enough and the faeces are dry and hard. It is usual to empty the bowel every day but for some people, twice a day is normal, and for others, once every two days is lucky. It is important to establish regular habits of emptying the bowel. Constipation is often caused by a diet containing insufficient bulk (not enough fibre), but emotional factors may also produce this condition. Before you reach for the laxatives, remember dependence upon them is often irritating to the intestine and is not natural. I think it is far better to increase the dietary intake of plant foods. These act as natural laxatives, since they contain large amounts of fibre (cellulose and other indigestible carbohydrates), which provide bulk that distends and stimulates the large intestine to function normally.

Diarrhoea (another one of those words which I hate trying to remember how to spell!) is a condition in which the faeces are very soft or watery and there is need to empty the bowel frequently. That is putting it politely! The problem is often caused by eating something which irritates the lining of the alimentary canal or by some infection. It is usually not serious but if it persists for more than a day or two, try fasting for 24–36 hours, resume your food intake again beginning with fruit and see how you go. In babies, diarrhoea can be serious because of the loss of water involved. Both constipation and diarrhoea can be caused by emotional upsets, certain medicines or an excess of certain foods. If at any time you have blood in your faeces, you should immediately seek help from a reliable practitioner.

THE WHY OF GOOD NUTRITION

Not many people could be said to be truly 'alive' at this moment. Change has never been easy for us, and we have always had to be prodded quite hard by nature before we would do much about it. Westerners are being ravaged by degenerative diseases on a scale that we have never seen before. We are eating ourselves to death! The way we treat our fellow creatures that share this planet with us reveals that we are still in the belief that all other life forms are basically second-class and only matter if they amuse us or make themselves useful to us.

Science fiction writers are warning us about visitors from other planets. I believe there are people from other worlds. They are watching us and saying to themselves, "There is no way I'm going to live on Earth until these earthlings get their act together. Look at what they eat!" Yes, these folks from other worlds are just waiting for us to go back to nature!

If you have been reading this book from the introduction to this page, then you would be informed about the value of living food and why you should eat raw, vitamins and minerals, detoxification, fasting and human digestion.

Before we go into the recipes, I would like you to consider the reason why we nourish ourselves in the first place. I would like you to consider the power within your blood. I guess you never thought of it that way before. I certainly didn't think much about it until I began to educate myself about nutrition.

We have sixty trillion cells in our body. Every cell lives for a limited time before it reproduces itself and dies. Every three months we get a new bloodstream, every eleven months each cell in our body has been renewed and every two years we get a new bone structure. Do you realise that by eating correctly for approximately two years, you could have a whole new body? You could be a totally new you. Isn't that encouraging? Doesn't it make you more aware of the

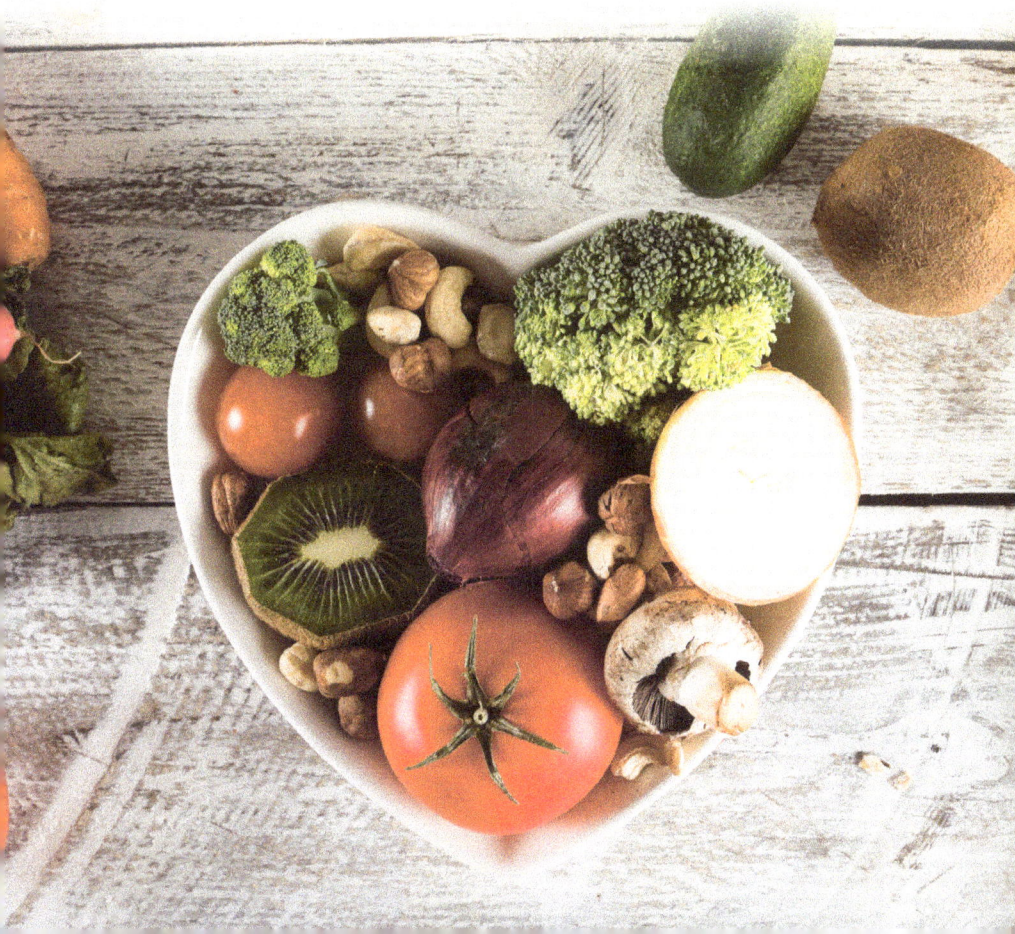

importance of the ingredients that you use, to make your body what it is today. *Remember: "What you eat and drink today, walks and talks tomorrow!"*

Clean, fresh, good food means a clean, fresh, good bloodstream. This means personal discipline and control on your part. How are you feeding your 60 trillion cells? The human body can take years of punishment before it rebels against being loaded down with valueless foods and the toxic poisons they produce. When the body cannot undo the damage done to it fast enough, the bloodstream becomes clogged and dirty. Then the whole system begins to break down and becomes a breeding ground for disease, which results in premature ageing. This does not have to happen. *We were created to live until we die, not dying the whole time that we are alive.*

I believe that good nutrition can help to reduce crime, empty the mental hospitals, contribute to a happy marriage or relationship with a friend and generally make us better people. A marriage has got to suffer if both partners are chronically fatigued and plagued with aches, pains, constant sickness and depression, as opposed to being healthy, strong and clear-minded. There are certain mental disorders that can definitely be relieved by a high raw diet, not to mention how many crimes or abuses could be avoided.

People carry between 10kg and 40kg of toxic poisons and wastes inside of them. If all those poisons don't get out, our body breaks down under the stress, we become sick and personal relationships are affected. There are many books written about the subject of crime and its relationship to food, but I don't see many authorities utilising the information, nor do I hear about people who embrace a back-to-basics-diet and -lifestyle committing crimes or acts of violence. If you have then I would like to know about it.

You might be thinking, "Hang on a second. Is Anne trying to tell us that if we all become vegetarian, eat raw foods and meditate that we will never commit acts of violence, rob a bank, get angry or divorce our family?" No...I am only trying to say that, in general, a healthy body leads to a productive, healthy mind. I still get cross or angry, and I still want to throw something at my husband sometimes, but when I get these urges I seem to be in more control these days and I calm down quickly. There is no need to get upset about things because things are usually not that important anyway. Important things are like when you find out you have cancer or you only have one day to live. That's when you can get upset if you wish, but only for an instant, because to be angry or upset is wasting precious time that you could spend being happy and free. Remember, there will always be someone else who is a lot worse off than you.

Now, let's look at some recipes!

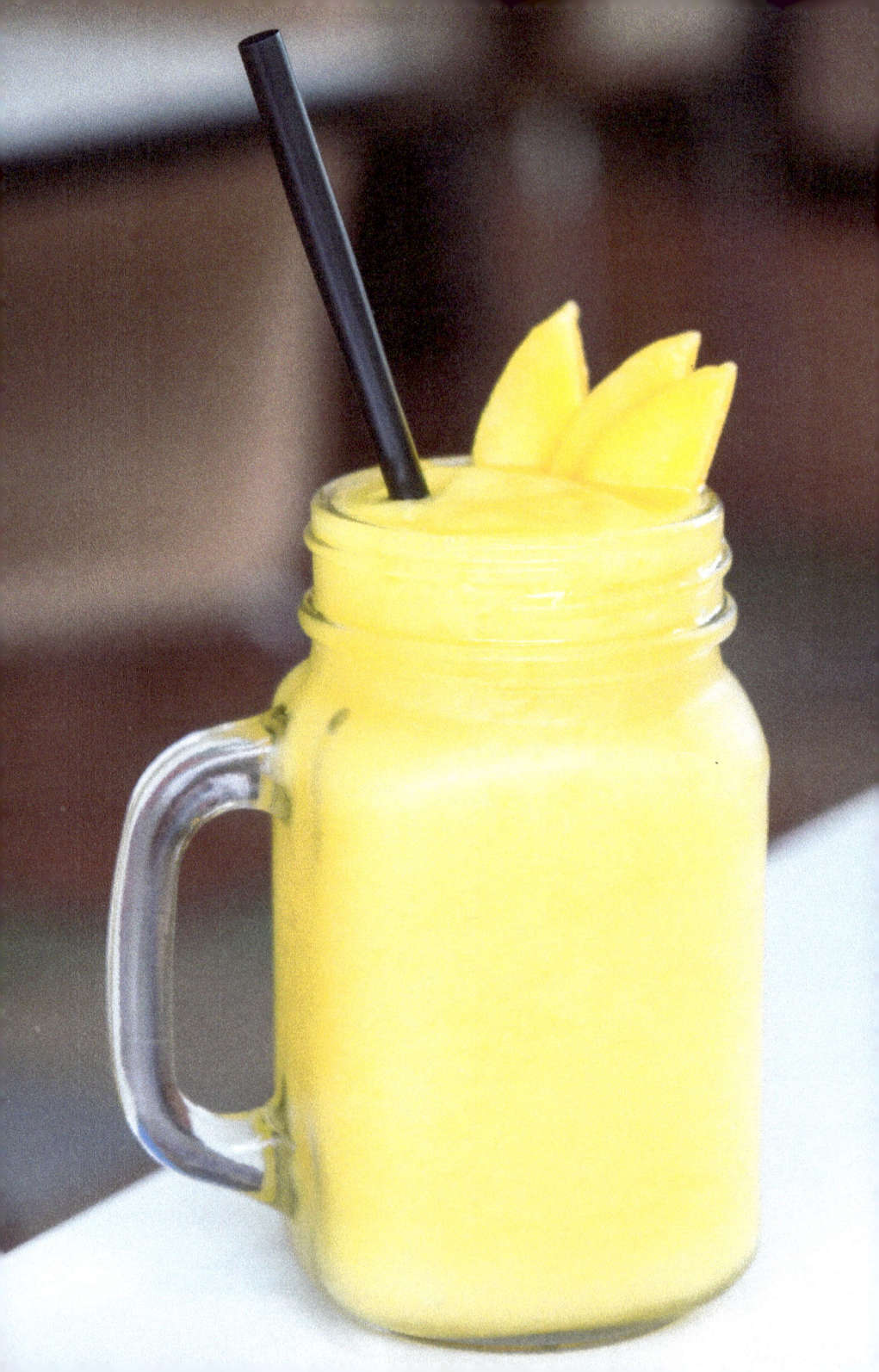

Recipes for Life

Fruit whip ideas

Fruit whip can be eaten at any time of the day. With the addition of seeds and nuts it can be transformed into a main meal. You may use a variety of fruits, the best being banana, mango, custard apple, black sapote, passionfruit, pawpaw, strawberries, plums and peaches. Simply change around the combinations until you are happy.

Fruit should be sliced into small pieces and placed in a container and frozen for at least 24 hours or until quite solid. Remove the fruit and place in a food processor or run through a Champion juicer with the homogenising plate in. It comes out like ice cream. Use no more than three fruits at one time.

Banana Mango Whip

Serves 3

2 bananas, sliced and frozen	1. Blend bananas first, then add mango pieces.
2 mangoes, sliced and frozen	2. While blending, add passionfruit pulp.
1 passionfruit, pulp only	3. Scrape out mixture and serve in chilled bowls with a sprinkle of sesame seeds for decoration and extra nutritional benefits.

Bananas – high in potassium

Anne Clark

Peach Whip

Serves 4

- 2 large peaches, sliced and frozen
- 5 large bananas, sliced and frozen
- 1 tbsp carob powder
- 1 tsp vanilla extract
- ¼ tsp cloves or nutmeg, ground

1. Blend all ingredients.
2. Chill, and serve with grated fresh coconut or lightly toasted sunflower seeds.

Ideal for the weight watcher

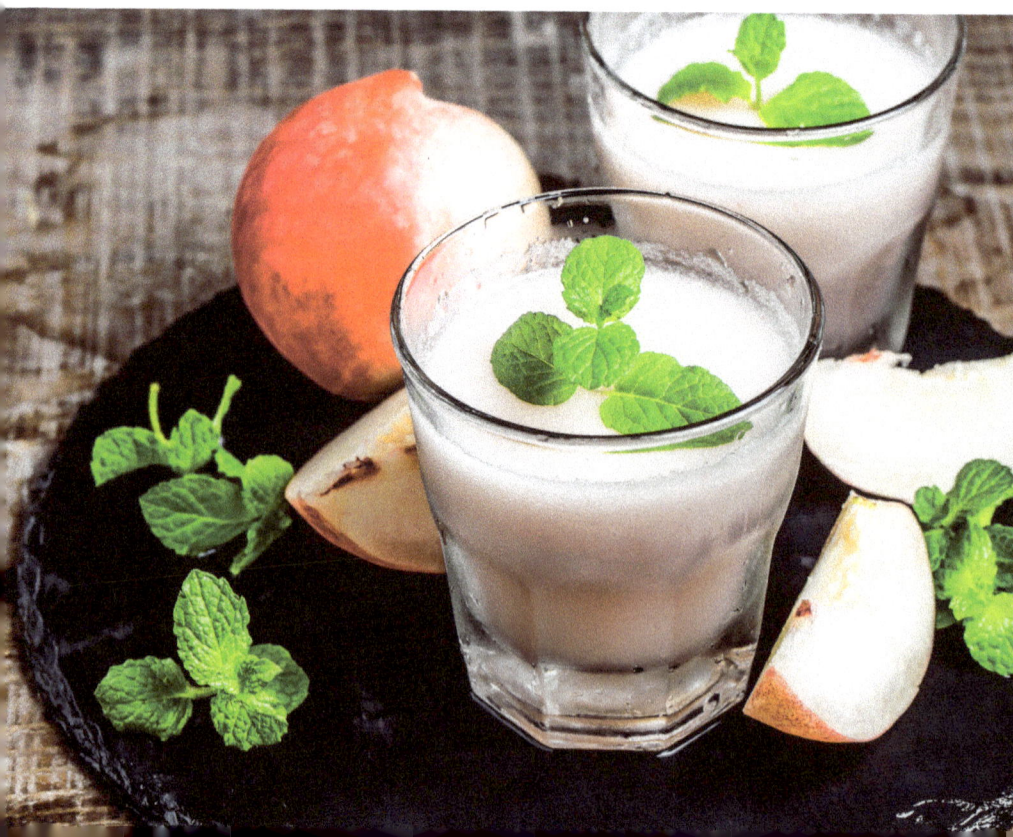

Fruit Cup

Serves 2

1 cup seedless grapes

1 cup peach, peeled and diced

1 cup raspberries or strawberries

Honey to taste

1. Blend with a little honey and serve in glass bowls or sherbet glasses.

Contains vitamin A and C… ideal for sickness recovery

Sunflower Whip

Serves 3

½ cup sunflower seeds

1–2 cups pawpaw, cubed

1 apple, chopped finely

1 cup pineapple pieces

2 tbsp pineapple juice

½ cup strawberries or other berries

1. Process ingredients in blender until smooth.
2. Serve chilled with a sprinkle of freshly grated coconut. You could also freeze this as a fruit sauce or to use as a filling for fruit puddings.

High protein
Digestive aid

Anne Clark

Prune Whip

This makes a creamy, rich dessert or breakfast treat. Add honey, nuts or cereal for variety.

Serves 3

- 1 cup dried prunes
- 250 g tofu or 1 cup diced banana pieces
- ⅓ cup pecans or walnuts, coarsely chopped
- 2 tbsp honey
- ½ cup prune juice (from cooked prunes)
- ¼ cup linseed (soaked in ½ cup water for one hour before use)

1. Place the prunes in a small bowl. Cover and soak overnight.*
2. Combine tofu or banana in a food processor with nuts, drained prunes and honey and blend, using a spatula to scrape down the sides between blending.
3. Add the prune juice and blend a little more.
4. Drain the linseed and reserve the juice.*
5. Add the linseed to prune whip and blend in well.
6. Serve the prune whip straight away in chilled bowls. Freeze for later use.

Gentle laxative

*Note: Use the linseed juice and the dried prune soaking water as a valuable addition to smoothie drinks and as a mild laxative drink. Tofu adds nutritional value to this whip, but if you would prefer not to use it, banana will make an acceptable replacement provided you use the whip straight away. Quite by accident I forgot to drain the prunes and linseed and blended them up with other ingredients. The result was quite satisfactory and I was able to transform the whip into a fruit sauce, dressing or icing for a fruit pie or cake. Add more liquid if you require a sauce-like consistency.

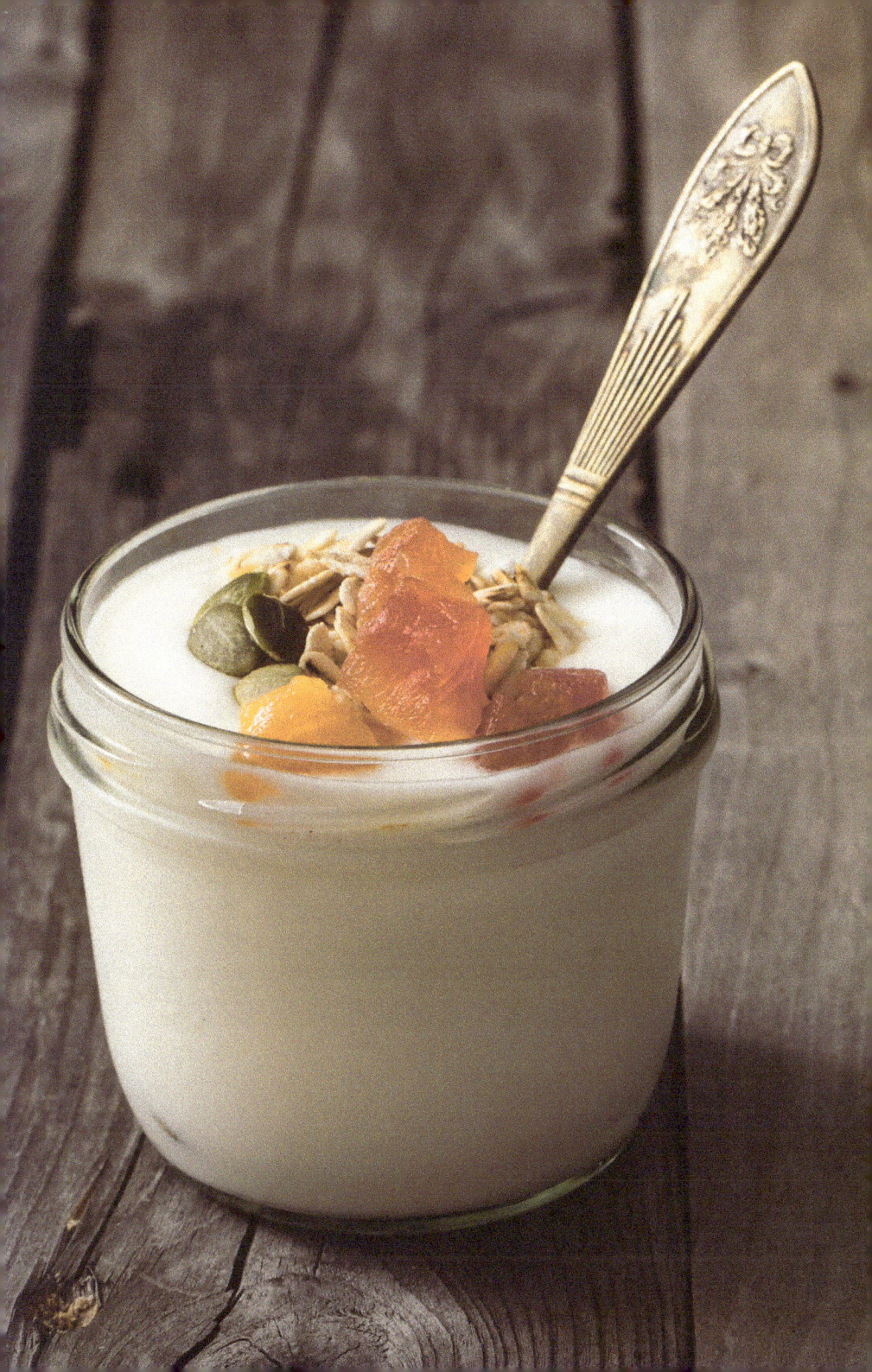

Anne Clark

Paradise Whip

This whip is more like an ice cream, and it is very rich so you only need a small amount. We have paradise whip for a lunchtime treat or dessert.

Serves 4

1 cup toasted cashew nuts (raw is better)

Blend until the cashew nuts become a fine meal, then add:

¼ cup dates, chopped

3 tbsp carob powder

5 large bananas, partly frozen, sliced

2 tbsp honey

1 tsp vanilla essence

2 custard apples, sliced into pieces

2 mangos, sliced into pieces

1. Blend the cashew nuts to a fine meal.
2. Place the above ingredients in a food processor in the listed order, then process until you are happy with the consistency.
3. Scrape out enough for intended serve and serve in a chilled bowl. Freeze the remaining whip for later use. For a softer serve, leave to thaw on kitchen sink for 10–15 minutes, depending on climate, then enjoy.

Dairy free and protein enriched

In the Raw

Banana Passionfruit Ice Cream Whip

Serves 6

- 1 tbsp sultanas
- ⅔ cup water
- 1⅓ cups soy milk powder (optional)
- 2 tsp lemon juice
- 2 large bananas, mashed
- 1 tsp vanilla essence
- 4 egg whites, stiffly beaten
- ⅔ cup passionfruit pulp (about 10 passionfruit)

1. Blend sultanas and water together.
2. Blend sultana mixture, soy milk powder, lemon juice, banana and vanilla until fluffy.
3. Transfer mixture to an electric mixer and add beaten egg whites and passionfruit. If you don't have an electric mixer, fold the mixture in by hand and mix well.
4. Pour into shallow trays and freeze.

This recipe does not require a second beating. Any fruits may be substituted for bananas and passionfruit. Egg whites can be left out of the recipe but expect a different texture.

Magnesium regulates acid-alkaline balance

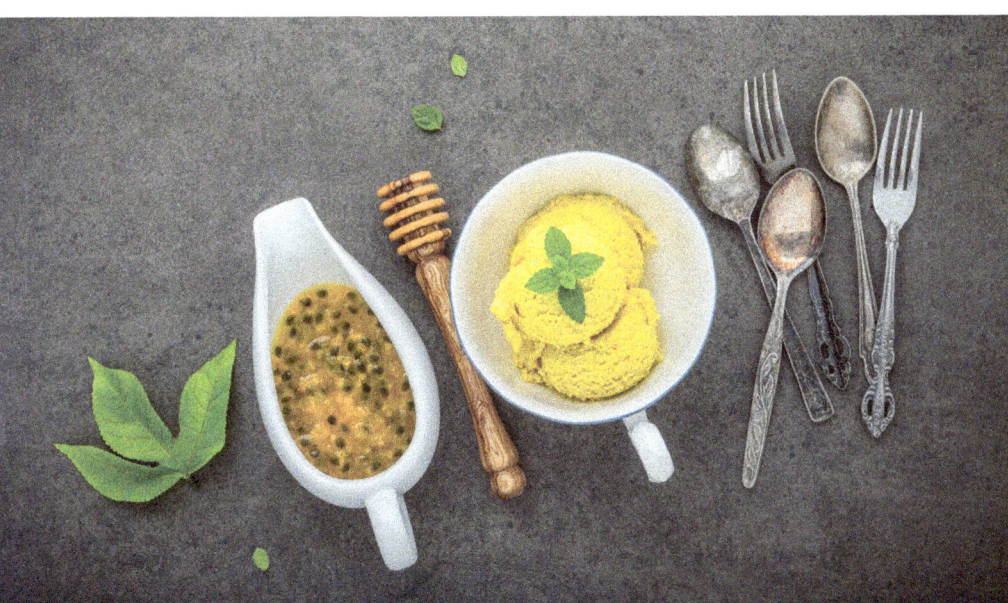

Liquid Breakfast

Breakfast is an important meal when it comes to balancing metabolism. It should be a reward for some sort of physical movement in the morning like walking, yoga or stretching. If you don't have much time for eating then these quick liquid breakfast ideas should do the trick. The following recipes are ideal for any time of the day, but your brain will utilise the nutrition more effectively if you serve these drinks as a breakfast.

The Grape Whammy

Grapes are a uniquely nourishing, strengthening, cleansing, regenerative food, useful in convalescence, for anaemia and fatigue, and for disorders such as arthritis, gout and rheumatism, which may result from poor elimination. Grapes should be eaten on their own, not as part of a meal, as they ferment rapidly in the stomach. Chewing grapes is also recommended for infected gums.

If you are not in the comfort of your own home, alternatively just buy a small bag of grapes and eat them until you are satisfied.

Serves 2–3

250 g fresh grapes, washed well

1 cup grape juice (chilled)

1. Blend well and sip slowly.

Skin tonic and detoxifier

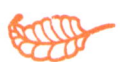

In the Raw

Rock 'n' roll

You may like to prepare this when you first rise in the morning. Go about your business, exercise, shower, etc., and then take time to enjoy this delight. Eat slowly and make sure you allow time to digest this breakfast. You can also puree the lot and serve as a cream.

Serves 3

- ½ apple, diced
- 2 tbsp sunflower seeds
- ½ peach, diced
- 1 tbsp sesame seeds
- 1 small banana, sliced
- 3 tbsp raisins
- 3 pitted dates, chopped finely
- Wheatgerm, sprinkle (optional)
- Soy milk or apple juice to cover

1. Mix fruits and seeds in a medium-sized bowl.
2. Sprinkle with wheatgerm.
3. Add milk or juice to moisten.
4. Let stand for a few minutes before serving.

Peaches are high in vitamin A, zinc and iodine

Fibre enriched

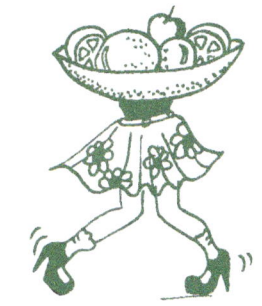

Anne Clark

Quick start shake

Serves 2

- 2 cups soy milk
- 1 tsp brewer's yeast
- 1 tsp carob powder
- 1 tsp kelp powder
- 1 tbsp almond butter
- 30 g alfalfa sprouts (optional)
- 2 tbsp honey
- 1 tsp lecithin granules

1. Combine ingredients in an electric blender and process at high speed until smooth.
2. Serve at breakfast or as a quick energy snack.

You may like to use fruit instead of, or as well as, carob powder.

Stress reliever

Slimming drink

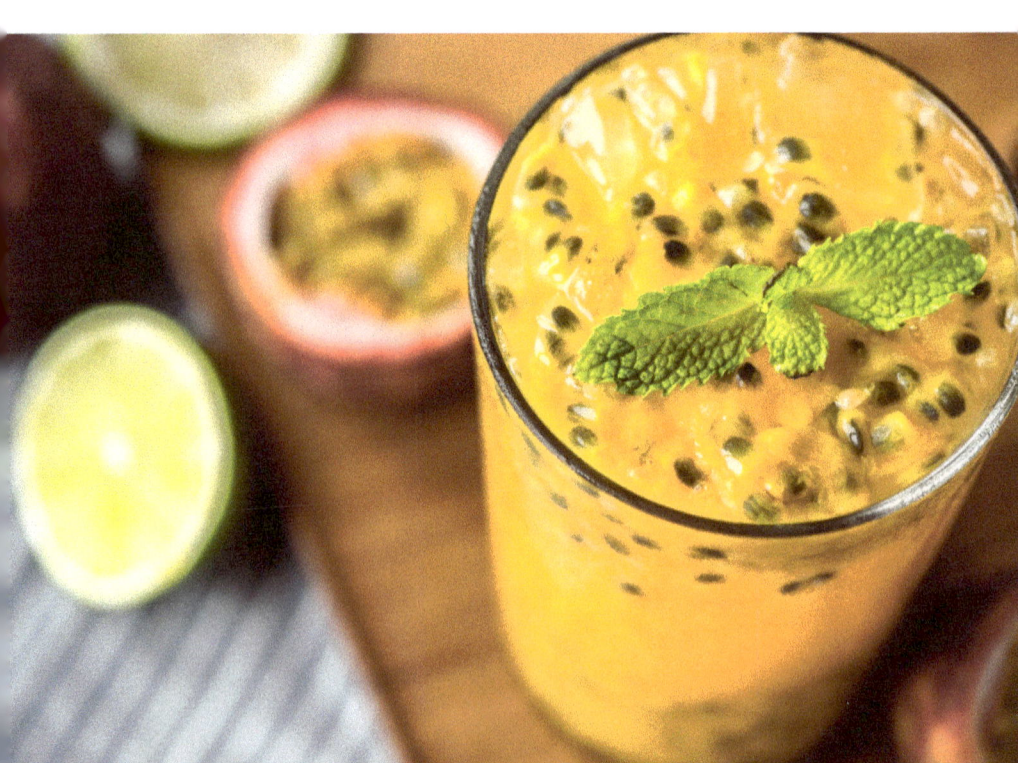

In the Raw

Happy Drink

Serves 1

1 cup fresh apple juice

1 pear

1. Simply blend until you have a suitable texture and drink.

Cleansing and purifying

The Mouth Spark

Serves 2

1 cup fresh pineapple

1 cup fresh orange juice

1 cup fresh grapefruit juice

1. Blend all ingredients and serve straight away.

Vitamin C enriched

Mango Passion Smoothie

Serves 2

1 medium ripe mango, peeled and chopped

1 cup soy milk or coconut milk

1 cup fresh apple juice

1 passionfruit, pulp only

1. Blend mango, milk and apple juice until smooth.
2. Stir in passionfruit.
3. Refrigerate before serving.

Mango is very high in vitamin A and great for skin

Mango allergy is common so be careful of the sap

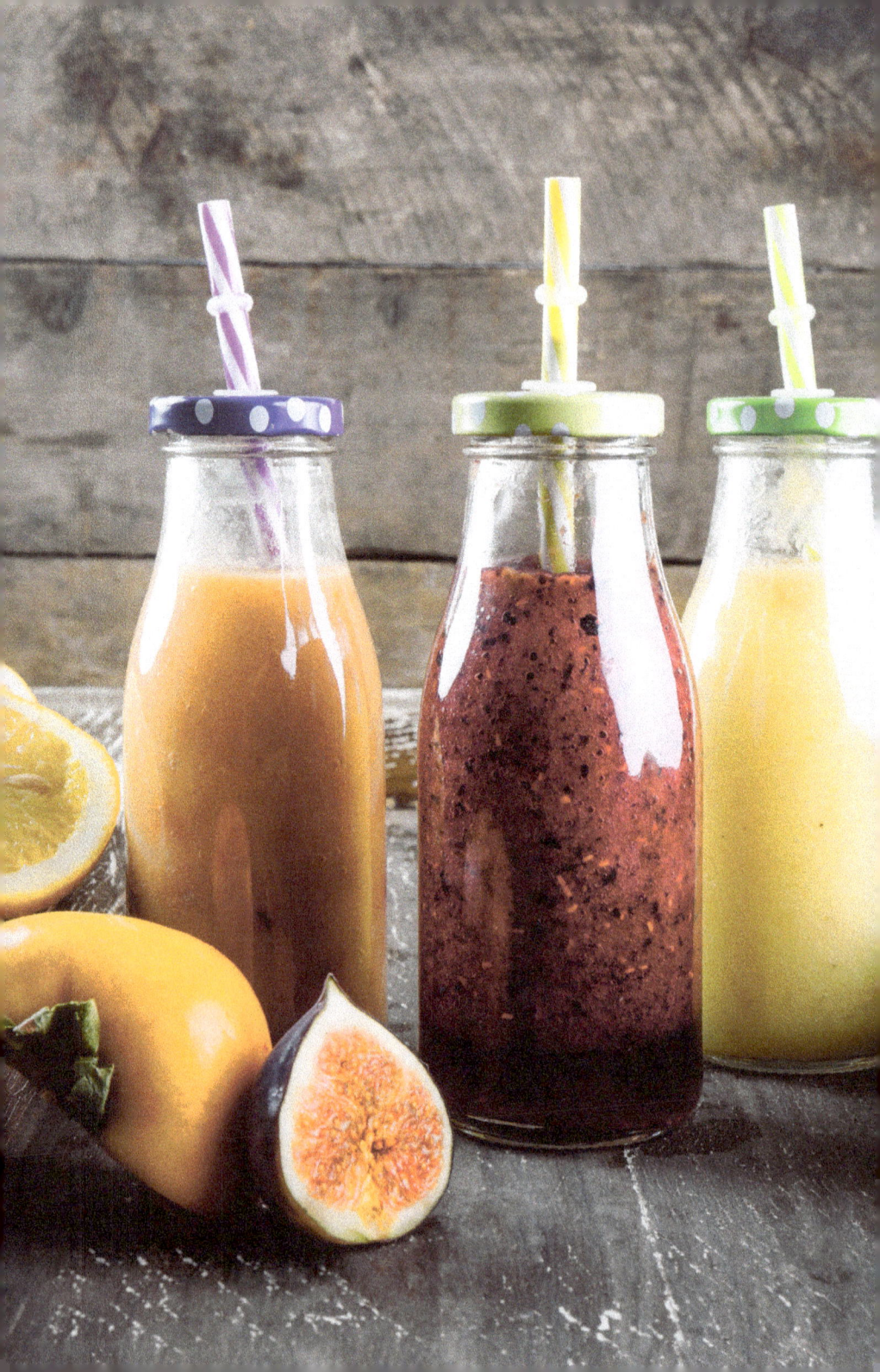

Beverages

No one can deny that fresh juices are so tempting and wonderful, yet how many of us indulge in freshly squeezed juice on a regular basis. If you haven't got a juicing machine, then go out and buy one. If you can't afford it, then sell the couch, sell anything, but get one! You can have a juice day once a week as part of a body cleanse or have a pre-dinner cocktail (carrot and celery with parsley) or start the day with a fresh fruit juice, which in turn could be your breakfast.

The various juice combinations are endless and I would need to write another book on the benefits of fresh juices in your diet, so I will simply pass on a few great combinations, which you may have already tried and some new ones you may have never thought of.

Apple and Orange Velvet

Serves 2

1 cup orange juice

1 tbsp lemon juice

1 cup apple juice

1 tbsp tofu or fruit puree

1. Process ingredients in an electric blender until smooth.

Vitamin C

Internal cleanser

Apple Pear Juice

Serves 2

1 cup apple juice

1 cup pear juice

1 passionfruit, pulp only

nutmeg, sprinkle

1. Blend fruit juice with passionfruit pulp.
2. Serve in chilled glasses with a sprinkle of nutmeg.

High folic acid alleviates constipation

Pineapple Crush

Serves 2-3

1 medium pineapple, chopped in small pieces

ice cubes

1. Place pineapple in blender with ice cubes.
2. Blend and serve.

Pineapple = manganese to aid memory

Carrot and Celery Cocktail

Serves 2-3

340 g carrots, washed and peeled

4 stalks celery

small bunch parsley

several lettuce leaves

1. Feed the carrots into the juicer first then follow with remaining vegetables.
2. Make sure the juice is well stirred before serving.

Cleanser for skin and blood

In the Raw

Apple Cordial

Serves 6

- 4 cups apple juice, chilled
- 12 whole cloves
- ½ cup honey
- 1 tsp ground nutmeg
- 6 lemon slices
- 6 cinnamon sticks

1. Combine all ingredients except cinnamon sticks and let stand for one hour.
2. Sieve the apple mixture into six mugs. Add cinnamon sticks for stirring.

Apples are the best fruit source of vitamin E for healthy muscles and nerves

Protects respiratory system from the poisons of city air

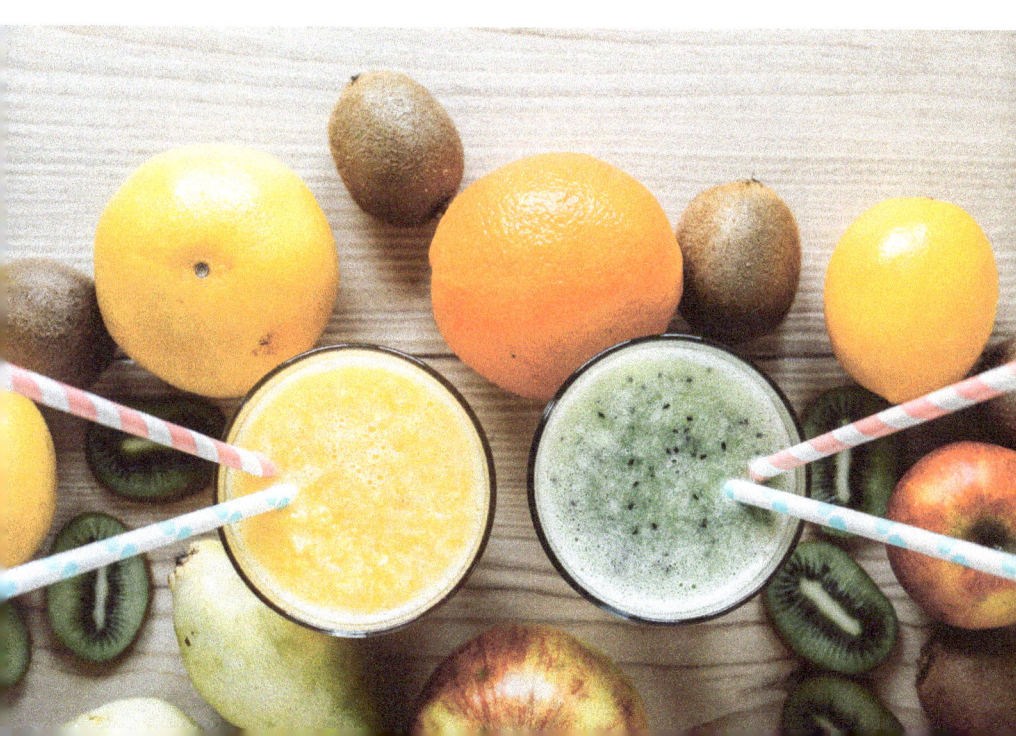

Anne Clark

Avocado Surprise

Serves 3-4

2 cucumbers, peeled and cut into chunks

½ lemon, juice (or lime)

½ ripe avocado, peeled

1 tsp vanilla essence (optional)

1. Process ingredients in an electric blender until liquefied.

Improves skin and nails

Brain Smoothie

Serves 1

¼ cup raisins, chopped finely

¼ cup almonds, ground

1 cup water

1 tbsp soy milk powder

1 tsp lecithin

1. Process ingredients in an electric blender until liquefied.

Note: The sediment of the raisins and almonds will fall to the bottom, so eat with a spoon or reserve for fruit whips, etc.

High in B3

Good for students

Super Drinks

There are drinks that you can whip up for an energy lift as well as for specific healing purposes. The following recipes contribute to your wellbeing and just happen to taste great too!

The Biotin Smoothie

Serves 2

- ¼ cup frozen mango pieces or alternative fruit
- 1½ cups soy milk or apple juice
- ¼ cup ground almonds
- 2 tsp lecithin granules
- 1 egg yolk
- 2 tsp honey
- 2 tsp brewer's yeast
- nutmeg, sprinkle

1. Blend all ingredients well, except for nutmeg.
2. Serve in chilled glasses with a sprinkle of nutmeg.

Stress reliever

High in B vitamins, calcium & magnesium

Great brain food!

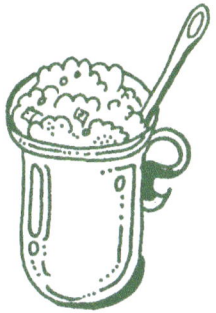

Anne Clark

Energy Lift Smoothie
Serves 2

For this recipe I suggest almond milk. To make the milk, grind 1½ cups almonds in a food processor. Add four cups water and some vanilla essence (optional). Blend well. Strain and serve. You can use other nuts instead of almonds. Keep the strained nut pieces and use for other recipes.

- 2 cups almond milk
- 1 tbsp tahini or peanut paste
- 1 tbsp honey
- 1 tbsp ground sunflower seeds
- 2 tsp wheatgerm
- 1 frozen banana, sliced
- 2 tbsp lecithin granules
- 1 tsp ground cinnamon

1. Put all ingredients in the blender and process thoroughly.
2. Serve in chilled glasses.

High calcium

Lemon-Limeade Smoothie

Serves 4-5

Ingredients	Instructions
3 tbsp honey	1. Combine honey and half of the hot water in an electric blender until the honey is dissolved.
1 cup hot water	
3 limes, juice of	2. Add the remainder of the water, juices and rinds.
1 grapefruit, juice of	
2½ cups water	3. Refrigerate until well chilled.
½ lemon, rind	4. Remove the rinds and serve over crushed ice, garnished with mint sprigs.
½ lime, rind	
3 lemons, juice of	
sprigs of mint to garnish	

Vitamin C

High fibre

Useful for treating colds and flu

Date Shake

Serves 2

Ingredients	Instructions
1 cup almond milk or alternative	1. Process ingredients thoroughly in an electric blender.
4 almonds, ground	2. Chill and serve.
1 cup apple juice	
4 ice cubes	
12 dates, pitted	
1 tsp. carob powder	

High magnesium

Nerve tonic

Tropical Madness

Serves 3-4

1 pineapple, rind removed, cut into chunks

½ cup pawpaw pieces, frozen

¼ small coconut, cut into pieces

coconut water (optional)

2 oranges, juice of

1–2 cups of ice cubes

1. Process pineapple flesh and pawpaw in an electric blender to liquefy.
2. Add orange juice, as well as coconut flesh and coconut water, if using. Process until smooth.
3. Add ice and process until ice is finely crushed. Serve at once.

Almost a headache cure

Fatigue Rescue

Serves 1

2 tbsp sesame seeds

3–4 almonds

1 tsp honey

1–2 cups water

½ tsp cinnamon

1 tsp vanilla essence

1. Put the sesame seeds and almonds in the blender with honey and a little of the water. Blend or process to a thick creamy paste.
2. Add the rest of the water, vanilla and cinnamon, and blend to a creamy milk.
3. Drink at once or use on your cereal.

Calcium enriched

In the Raw

What's in a Cup Berry Juice

Serves 1-2

1 cup strawberries

1 cup raspberries

1 cup red grape juice

mineral water

1. Puree strawberries and raspberries in a blender or food processor until smooth.
2. Add grape juice.
3. Dilute with mineral water if necessary.

These fruits combined = blood purifier

High fibre

Small amount of calcium & phosphorus

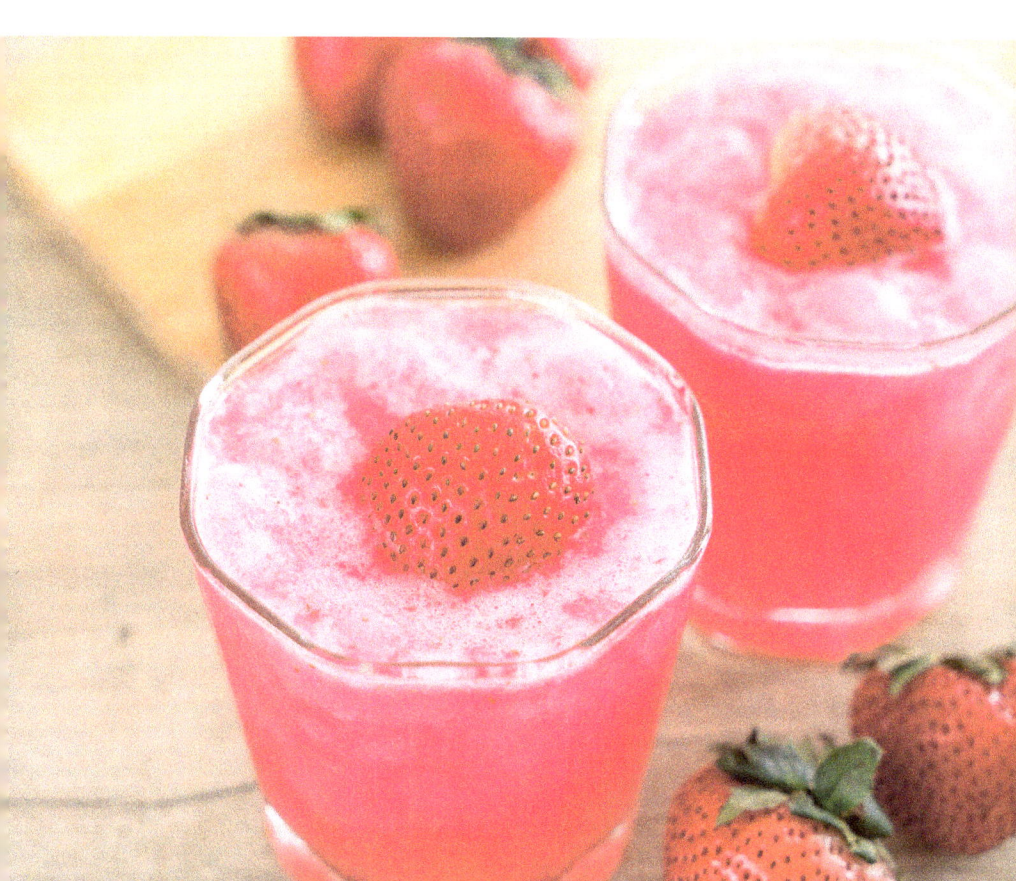

Anne Clark

Nut Milk Shake

Serves 2

30 g cashew nuts, ground

1 cup almond milk or water

3 bananas, sliced

¼ tsp kelp powder

1. Liquefy the cashew nuts with the almond milk or water in a blender.
2. Add remaining ingredients and process until smooth.

Calcium and potassium enriched

Runner's Lift Shake

Serves 2

2 cups coconut milk

1 tsp honey

1 tbsp tahini (sesame seed paste)

2 tbsp wheatgerm or oats

1 egg yolk (optional)

1 tsp carob powder

1. Process ingredients in a blender until smooth.

Recovery and energy tonic

In the Raw

Breakfasts For Busy People

Pawpaw with Snow

Serves 1

½ medium pink pawpaw

coconut, freshly grated

1. Peel and chop pawpaw into bite-sized chunks and place in a bowl.
2. Sprinkle freshly grated coconut over the pawpaw.
3. Mix through if you wish and eat with delight.

High in vitamin A and vitamin C

Good for skin

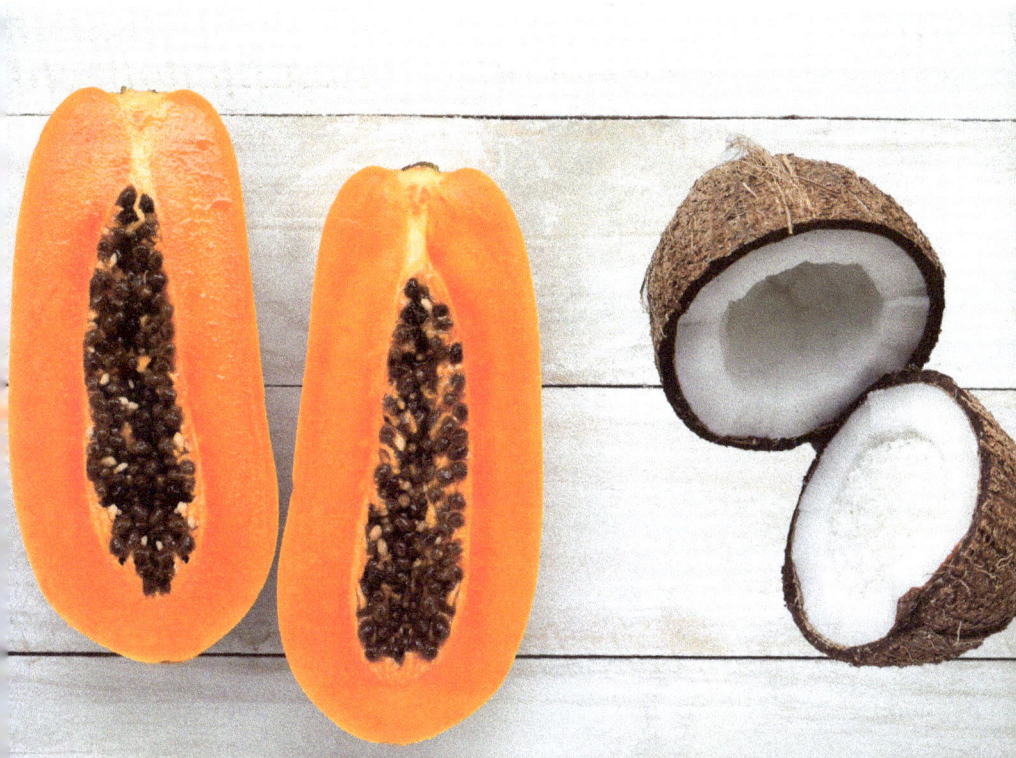

Anne Clark

Fruit Salad

Serves 2-3

Quite often people ask me, "What do I give my kids for breakfast as an alternative to cereal or toast?" It may be an obvious answer to most of you, but for those who have never considered fruit salad, the following recipe will be a treat to your children and adults alike. If the morning is always a rush, prepare the fruit the night before and store covered in the refrigerator. Remember some of the nutrients are lost in cutting and storage.

½ small pawpaw

½ small pineapple

6 dried figs, soaked (reserve the juice)

2 fresh apricots, plums or nectarines

1–2 passionfruit, pulp only

1 peach

1. Slice and cube the fruits.
2. Arrange in glass bowls so their gentle colours stand out (this is more attractive to children).
3. Scrape out the pulp of the passionfruit and combine with the reserved fig juice.
4. Pour over the fruit and serve at once.

Vitamin C and A

Pineapples are helpful with weight control and menstruation

In the Raw

Citrus Salad

Serves 2

1 orange, peeled

1 cup pineapple pieces

1 grapefruit, sliced

1–2 kiwi fruit

1. Arrange chopped citrus fruits in two medium-sized bowls.
2. Scoop out the flesh of kiwi fruit, then puree, blend or mash, and pour it over the citrus fruits.

Vitamin C   High fibre

Melon Salad

Serves 3-4

¼ honeydew melon

½ cantaloupe (also known as rockmelon)

¼ small watermelon

1. Cut the rinds off the melons and slice.
2. Arrange the slices on salad plates and serve chilled.

Aids weight loss

Blueberry Whip

Serves 2-3

1 cup blueberries

2 peaches

1–2 apples

1 apricot

1. Place peaches, apples and apricots in a food processor. Process just enough to break down fruit.
2. Remove the fruit and add blueberries.
3. Mix well. Serve in small glass bowls.

Zinc   Energy

ABC Mix

Serves 4

4 apples, grated

2 bananas, mashed

¼ cup chopped dates

½ cup shredded coconut

½ cup almond meal

1. Mix together the grated apples, bananas and dates.
2. Add coconut and almond meal slowly, cutting back on almond meal if necessary Mix to a pudding consistency.
3. Chill to eat the next day or use as a pie filling.

Laxative

Soaked Muesli

Serves 1

½ cup boiling water

3–5 tbsp oat flakes]

1 tbsp coconut yoghurt

1 lemon, juice of

1 apple

raw ground nuts

1. Mix water with oat flakes and soak overnight.
2. In the morning, add coconut yoghurt and the lemon juice.
3. Grate the apple with its peel over the mixture and sprinkle some raw, ground nuts on top.

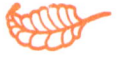

Breakfast For Lunch

The following recipes are traditionally consumed at breakfast, but for maximum digestion efficiency try eating them around lunch time.

Simple Breakfast Cereal

Serves 1

2 tbsp wheatgerm

1 tsp sesame seeds

1 banana, sliced

1 tsp honey or alternative sweetener

almond milk or soy milk to serve

1 small apple, chopped finely into cubes

1. Pour wheatgerm into a cereal bowl and sprinkle with sesame seeds.
2. Add banana and apple.
3. Sweeten to taste with honey or alternative.
4. Serve with almond or soy milk. Enjoy!

Rich in vitamin E and B-complex vitamins

Healthy cereal for children who do not eat enough food

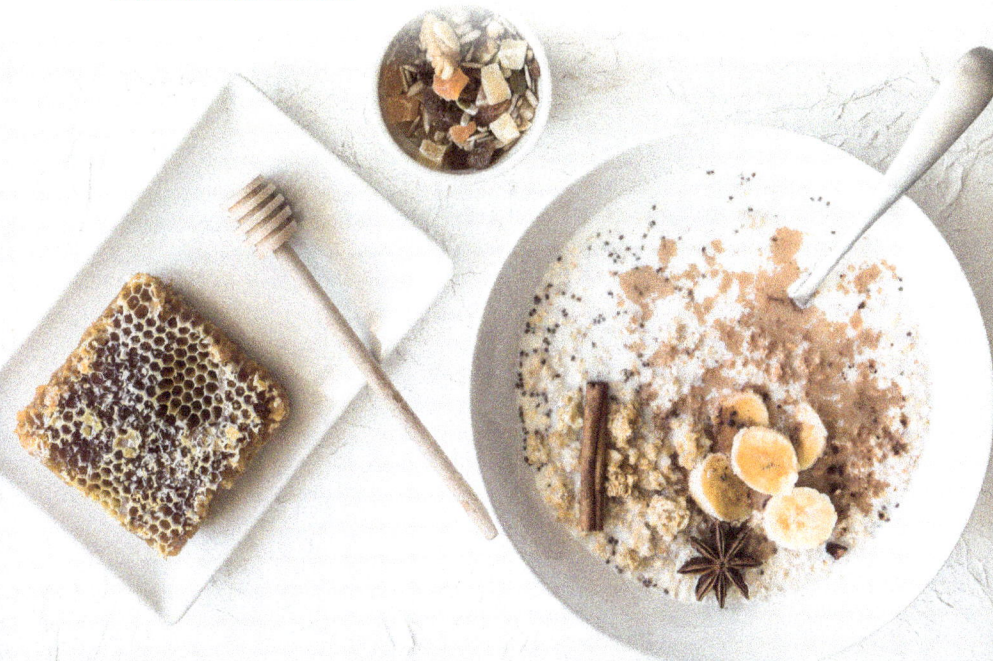

Anne Clark

Annie's Classic Midday Muesli

Serves 1

½ cup puffed rice cereal

¾ cups raw muesli (preferably organic)

1 tsp torula yeast powder

3 tsp lecithin granules

1 tsp liquid malt

3 chopped dried figs (pre-soaked)

¼ cup fig soaking juice or water

1 cup soy milk or apple juice

rice bran, sprinkle (optional)

apple, grated (optional)

1. Combine all ingredients in a medium-sized bowl. Allow to soak overnight in the refrigerator if possible or for at least one hour before consuming. Add more liquid to serve if necessary.

Ideal for safe weight gain

High in most vitamins and minerals

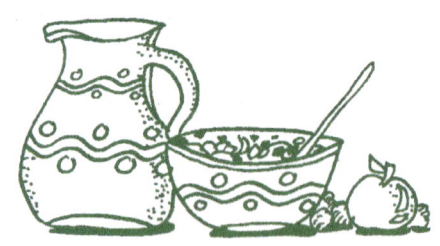

In the Raw

Salads

Salad dishes can be many and varied, and that is an understatement. Too often, the concept of a salad is merely a bowl of lettuce and tomato, very plain with little nutritional value, particularly when the amount eaten is a very small portion of a traditional meat-orientated meal. For starters, lettuce and tomato are the last ingredients I think of for a salad. Let us change the whole concept of a salad by making it the most important part of the meal and everything else is just extra.

Salads prepared creatively using the vast selection of vegetables and greens available and accompanied by living sprouts can become a nourishing main course or a substantial side dish to a lightly cooked

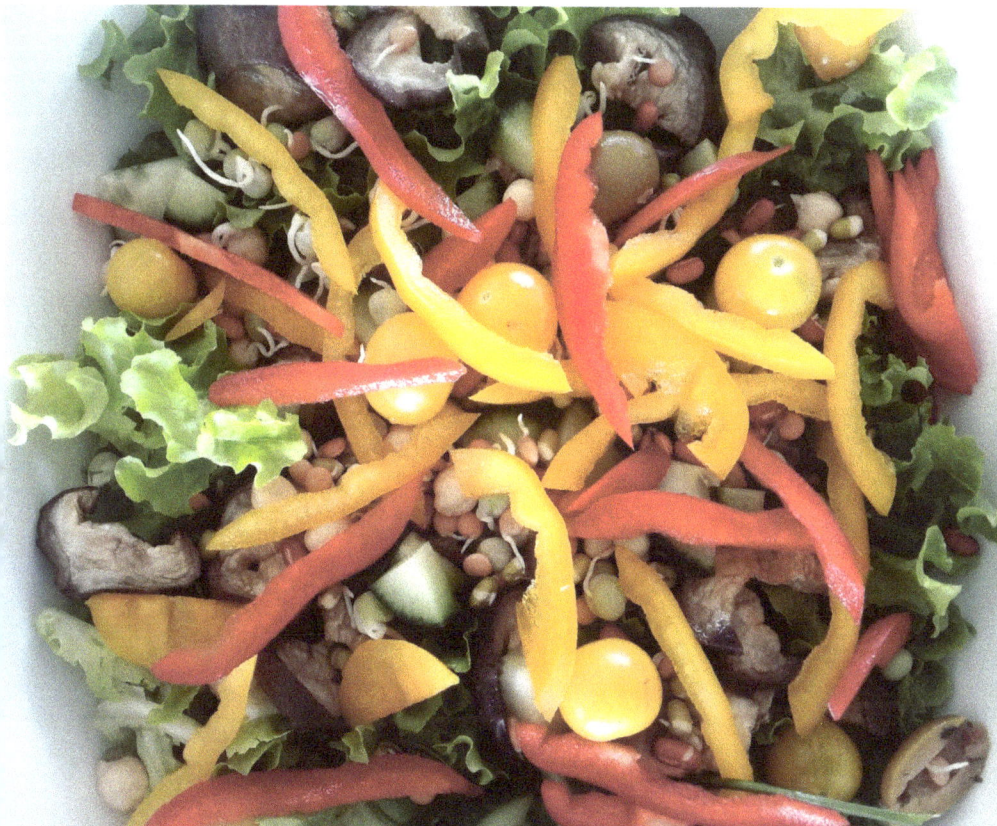

vegetarian main dish (for those who haven't discovered a 100% raw experience).

By now, we all know that to obtain the optimum nourishment from Mother Nature's abundant supply of natural fresh foods, it is best to eat them uncooked, unprocessed and preferably organically grown. In this form the enzymes, vitamins and minerals remain intact, while the life energy of the plant is also still present. In the case of dried seeds and beans, it is best to sprout rather than cook them.

Sprouting increases the vitamin content many times over, improves the protein by changing complex proteins to simple easily digestible amino acids and, most importantly, brings the seed to life, thus creating a living food. The life force in plants is a valuable source of nourishment, providing extra energy and enabling the body to become more vital. Since chlorophyll is such an important aspect of a healthy diet, it is a good idea to include plenty of fresh uncooked greens with any main meal.

Fruits are of course very cleansing especially to the digestive system and are best eaten at separate meals to vegetables or a little time prior to a main meal. There are some exceptions to this, such as apple, which seems to combine well with raw vegetables. You will notice that some of my salad dressing recipes have orange or lemon juice as an ingredient. Citrus juices actually enhance the salad and contribute to better digestion in most cases.

There are many types of salad greens including sprouts, herbs and vegetables. It is up to you to explore these wonderful living foods and incorporate them into your salads. Try using silverbeet, fennel, Chinese cabbage and endive instead of lettuce, and don't be afraid to eat cauliflower raw – it will make your salad more appetising and original.

Great Salad Ideas

The following recipes are simply guides and examples for you to follow. You may substitute ingredients where possible and alternate the dressings. You may also like to serve your salads as the main meal with interesting dips and celery, carrot and zucchini sticks. Actually, I like to spread one of my dips over a rice cake (which is one of the few cooked foods I eat) and top with salad and sprouts. You will discover your own preference. Whatever it is, remember to vary your salads every day and buy small amounts of vegetables at a time to keep control of freshness and cut down on waste.

Spinach & Mushroom Salad

Serves 2

This salad is rich in chlorophyll and iron and, with the addition of mushrooms, you get zinc as well. If you are fatigued, suffering from mental strain or stressed out, consider this salad as a positive force which will help to revitalise your body and mind.

1 small bunch of spinach or 3–4 leaves of silverbeet

6 mushrooms, sliced thinly

¼ cup pumpkin seeds

¼ cup chopped shallots

¼ cup fresh parsley, chopped finely

¼ cup alfalfa sprouts (optional)

1. Combine spinach with mushrooms, seeds, parsley and shallots.
2. Arrange sprouts around the salad.
3. Serve as is or with Oriental Dressing (see recipe), together with Savoury Balls or Vegetarian Pate (see recipe) and rice cakes.

Chlorophyll and magnesium

Anne Clark

Beetroot Side Salad

Serves 4

Beetroot juice is a powerful blood cleanser and tonic. It is useful for the treatment of anaemia and has the ability to enhance the immune system. Slimmers would do well to include beetroot in their diet, raw of course!

2 beetroots, scrubbed and trimmed

½ cup fresh parsley, chopped finely

2 tbsp fresh herbs, chopped finely

2 tbsp sesame seeds or chopped nuts

1. Shred fresh beetroot with fine grater or shredder. Mix in all other ingredients.
2. Toss with oil/lemon dressing if desired. Serve alongside greens and sprouts.

Beetroot juice can relieve menstruation troubles

Anne's Waldorf Salad

Serves 2-3

Celery has a strong effect on the kidneys and helps to eliminate wastes. It is rich in calcium and acts as an anti-inflammatory agent that clears uric acid from painful joints. Eat more celery for better digestion and even sexual stimulation. Apples also aid in digestion and they are rich in vitamin C and pectin which help to keep cholesterol levels stable. If you suffer from arthritis, rheumatism or gout this salad will be very beneficial.

1½ cups celery, sliced

1½ cups apple, chopped

¼ cup walnuts or almonds, chopped finely

1. Mix all ingredients well and place in a glass salad bowl.
2. Mix mayonnaise in with the salad.

Slimmer's delight

Sprouted Tabouli Salad

Serves 3

1 cup dried wheat, soaked 12 hours then sprouted 1-2 days

½ bunch parsley, finely chopped

¼ cup mint, finely chopped

⅓ cup lemon juice

1–2 tomatoes, finely chopped

¼ cup shallots, finely chopped

1 tsp olive oil

1. Combine all ingredients together in a mixing bowl. If desired, wheat can be chopped first in food processor.
2. Serve as a delicious live food side salad.

Protein and iron enriched

Sprouted Mung Bean Salad

Serves 3-4

We already know what a wonderful source of vitamins and minerals sprouted seeds are, but consider the boost they give in metabolising fats and oils and the added bonus they have of being pollution and chemical free!

2 cups sprouted mung beans

2 cups corn kernels

1. Combine sprouts and corn in a medium-sized salad bowl. Serve with other salads.

Protein enriched

Tomato, Mushroom and Basil Salad

Serves 4

4 lettuce leaves	1. Line a serving bowl with lettuce.
Alfalfa sprouts, handful	2. Place alfalfa, mushrooms, tomatoes and spring onions in a bowl.
Mushrooms, handful	3. Combine the basil with a dressing of your choice and pour over the salad.
4 medium tomatoes, sliced	4. Spoon the mixture into the serving bowl lined with lettuce.
½ bunch spring onions, sliced	*Chlorophyll, iron and zinc*
½ small bunch basil (20 leaves approx.), chopped finely	

Watercress Salad

2 bunches of watercress	1. Chop everything up finely and add to the watercress.
½ small cabbage	2. Serve with the dressing of your choice.
1 green capsicum	*Cleansing and high in antioxidants*
1 onion	
1 stalk celery	

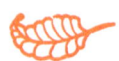

In the Raw

Nutty Pumpkin And Snow Pea Salad

Serves 6

Pumpkins are full of beta-carotene, the vitamin A precursor that helps protect us against cancer, heart troubles and respiratory disease. Snow peas are always expensive but don't let that stop you from adding them to salads.

500 g butternut pumpkin, grated

250 g snow peas

3 medium zucchini, sliced

½ cup pecan nuts, chopped finely or left whole (your choice)

1 tsp grated fresh ginger

1 tbsp honey

2 tbsp soy sauce

2 tbsp lemon juice

½ cup orange juice

1. Combine pumpkin, snow peas and zucchini in a bowl with the pecans.

2. Mix the remaining dressing ingredients together in a jar, then pour the dressing over the salad gradually, reserving some to use with other salads.

Vitamin A

Healthy skin and hair

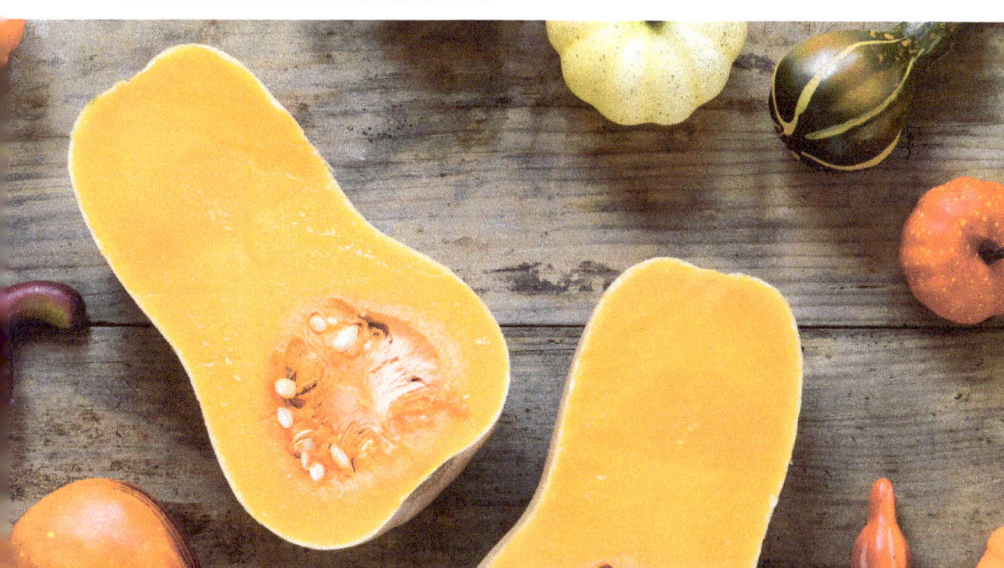

Anne Clark

Special Garden Salad

Serves 4

Usually I do not combine fruit with vegetables. For this salad I make the exception and, besides, it's all in the eating. Start by serving this salad as an entree and carefully picking out and eating all the fruit first. Wait a while before you start on the salad vegetables and you shouldn't have too much trouble digesting this delight. Good food deserves to be eaten slowly and therefore appreciated longer!

750 g snow peas, washed

6 mushrooms, thinly sliced.

dill or parsley, sprigs

½ punnet of raspberries, washed and drained

½ punnet of strawberries, washed & halved

1 orange or mandarin, peeled & segmented

1 small bunch grapes, washed & halved

½ punnet of cherry tomatoes, washed

assorted salad greens of your choice (e.g. radicchio, cos, butter, mignonette, watercress, endive)

1. Toss together all ingredients in a large bowl and pour over dressing of your choice.

   Silicon – the beauty mineral

In the Raw

Rootie-Tootie Salad

Serves 3-4

Turnips are recommended for gout in traditional medicine, as they are eliminators of uric acid. Carrots are rich in beta-carotene and are vital for building our resistance to respiratory infections and for disorder of the skin and eyes. Carrots are also up there with other vegetables as warriors against cancer, especially lung cancer. Eating carrots will increase levels of red blood cells. If you want to stay young, healthy and unwrinkled you should eat plenty of carrots.

1 large carrot

2 small turnips

1 celery stalk

1 medium beetroot

1 small bunch watercress

1 small sweet potato

1. Grate the carrot, turnips, beetroot and sweet potato, but keep the beetroot at a safe distance from other vegetables until you're ready for it.
2. Clean and trim the watercress.
3. Combine all the vegetables except the beetroot in a bowl.
4. Pour over dressing of your choice, toss gently, cover and chill for an hour or so.
5. Serve in small bowls with the grated beetroot on top.

Cleansing and slimming salad

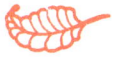

Anne Clark

Autumn Salad

Serves 4

Winter vegetables can be just as good raw and equally nutritious as summer vegetables. Broccoli is rich in vitamin C and iron. The anaemic, the fatigued and those with nervous problems should include iron in their diet.

1 cup broccoli, trimmed	1. Cut the broccoli into small spears, the fennel into thin strips, the turnips and carrots into round slices and the sprouts into quarters.
1 cup cauliflower pieces	
1 cup fennel, trimmed	2. Mix together in a large bowl with the cauliflower pieces.
½ cup turnip, scrubbed, peeled and grated	3. Pour Apple Tahini Dressing (see recipe) over the salad and mix thoroughly.
1 cup carrots, scrubbed or peeled	*Contains vitamins A & C and B-complex vitamins*
1 cup Brussels sprouts, trimmed	

In the Raw

Vegetable Platter

- 1 red capsicum
- 1 small beetroot
- 400 g broccoli flowerettes
- 400 g cauliflowerettes
- ½ cup slivered almonds
- 1 large carrot

1. Alternate broccoli and cauliflower on an oblong serving platter, leaving 4-5cm around the outer edge.
2. Arrange capsicum across broccoli and cauliflower.
3. Peel and slice beetroot and carrot and cut into thin long strips suitable to dip with. Place them in a separate bowl and sprinkle with slivered almonds.
4. Serve with a dressing in a small bowl beside the platter or spoon over vegetables.

Vitamin A & biotin, potassium and phosphorus.

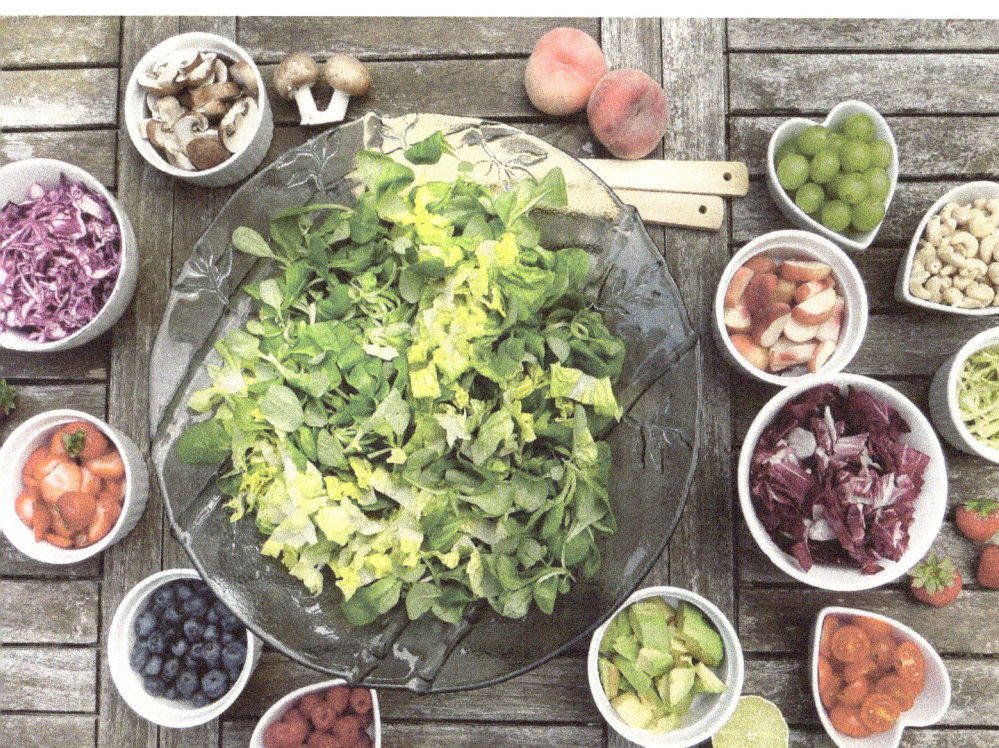

Anne Clark

Avocado Surprise Salad

Serves 2-3

Avocados are a complete food, supplying a little protein and starch as well as a pure oil which is mainly a monounsaturated fat. Rich in potassium, avocado therefore helps with fatigue, depression and poor digestion among other things. It is also a good source of vitamin A, some B-complex, a little C and some vitamin E. Women tend to avoid avocados because they think they will get fat, yet they are the same ones to tuck into a tub of yoghurt or consume low-fat cheeses. The fats in an avocado are much easier to digest, so do yourself a favour and choose avocados over dairy products; your skin will thank you!

2 medium avocados, cubed

1 tomato, cubed

1 cup corn kernels

1 capsicum, sliced finely

½ cup pine nuts

2 tbsp freshly chopped parsley

1. Combine all ingredients and add a little dressing.

Avocado helps your nerves

Luncheon Salad

Serves 4-5

1 cup alfalfa sprouts

1 cup fresh bean sprouts (e.g. mung or lentil)

2 cups shredded lettuce

1 capsicum, chopped

1 zucchini, sliced

1 carrot, grated

chives, freshly cut

red cabbage, small amount, sliced finely

1. Combine all ingredients and place in a medium-sized salad bowl.
2. Serve with a sprinkle of freshly grated coconut. This salad goes well with sprouted mung bean bread.

High digestive enzymes

Relieves stress

Green Salad

Serves 3-4

1 zucchini, sliced thinly

2 cups shredded lettuce

1 cup shallots, chopped

1 cucumber, sliced thinly

1 green capsicum, sliced thinly

1 avocado, peeled and cubed

fresh parsley, chopped

fresh chives, chopped

1. Combine all ingredients in a medium-sized salad bowl. Serve with Savoury Balls.

Chlorophyll = blood food

Dressings

A salad dressing should never overpower the actual salad. I can remember the traditional coleslaw salad swimming in mayonnaise served up in restaurants. That's fine if you want to eat mayonnaise, but I couldn't think of anything worse! Choose your dressings carefully and combine them with salad combinations that you know will be enhanced by the dressing rather than destroyed. Mix your dressings in jars and store the remainder of the dressing in the refrigerator for future use. Never keep dressings too long. Always smell them before using.

The following recipes are sure to give you more ideas and really stimulate your family and friends' appetite for more salads and less cooked foods!

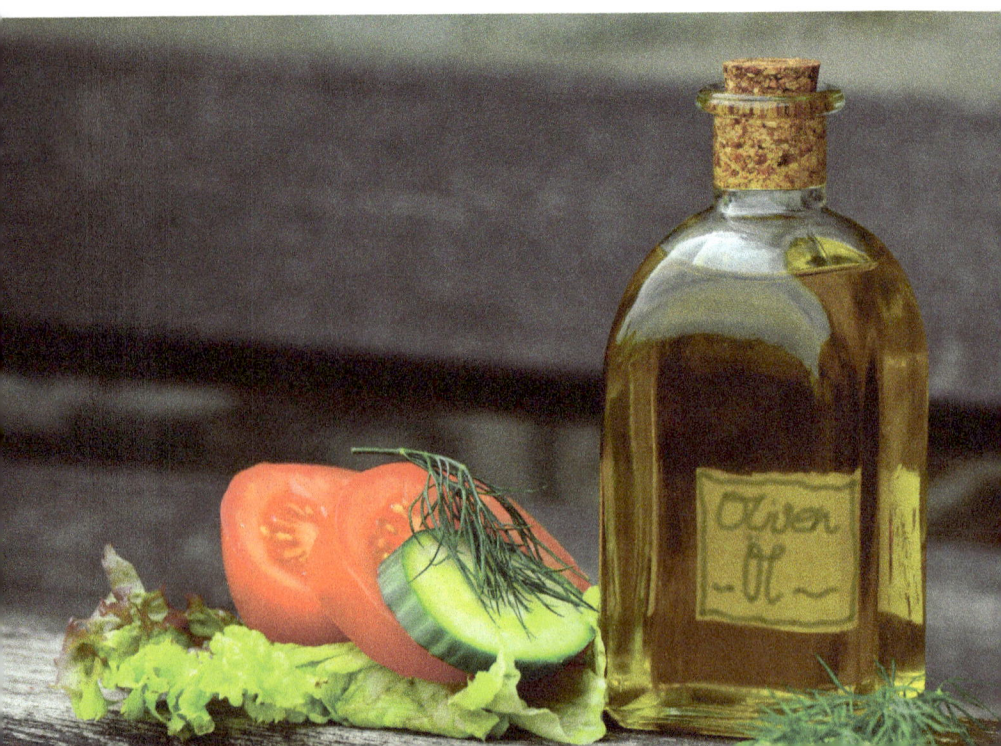

Apple Tahini Dressing

5 tbsp apple juice	1. Mix the apple juice gradually into the tahini.
2 tbsp tahini (sesame seed paste)	2. Add the remaining ingredients and season to taste.
1 tsp tamari (soy sauce)	*Good for constipation as fibre enriched*
1 tsp lemon juice	
1 drop dōTERRA Lemon essential oil	
¼ tsp black pepper	
1 drop dōTERRA Black Pepper essential oil	
Sprinkle of ground celery powder	

Walnut Dressing

- 125 g walnut pieces
- 2 cloves garlic
- ¼ tsp black pepper
- 1 tsp miso
- 2 tbsp olive oil
- 2 tbsp lemon juice
- ½ cup water

1. In a food processor, grind the walnuts with garlic and pepper.
2. Add the miso, olive oil and lemon juice and blend.
3. Add the water very gradually, blending continuously, until the dressing has the consistency of thick yoghurt. Use immediately.

Protein enriched

Traditional Mayonnaise

2 egg yolks (at room temperature)

240 ml sunflower oil

1 tbsp lemon juice

½ tsp mustard powder

1. Place egg yolks in a small warm bowl. Whisk lightly with a wire whisk or electric mixer at medium speed. Add a little oil gradually while whisking.
2. Add remaining oil and lemon juice with mustard powder and mix until well combined.
3. Put into a glass jar, cover and store in the refrigerator. The mayonnaise should keep for 4–6 weeks if stored properly.

High protein

Vitamin A

Cashew Mayonnaise

¾ cup ground raw cashew nuts

1 cup water

1 tsp kelp powder

1 tsp nutmeg, ground

2 tbsp lime or lemon juice

1. Add ground cashew nut meal to the food processor.
2. Add water and process until combined.
3. Add remaining ingredients and continue blending until mixture is creamy.
4. Keep blend in a well-sealed jar for 1–2 weeks in the refrigerator. Use instead of traditional mayonnaise.

Excellent protein balance

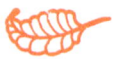

Oriental Dressing

1 cup orange juice

2 tbsp chopped fresh parsley

1 tbsp soy sauce (low salt)

1 tsp lemon juice

1. Combine all ingredients in a small jar and shake vigorously. Use within two days.

Vitamin C

High fibre

Clifton Dressing

Instead of French dressing I decided to name my dressing after Clifton Beach. Well, why not!

1 tbsp lemon juice

4 tbsp olive oil or alternative oil

2 spring onions, trimmed and finely chopped

1–2 cloves garlic, crushed

black pepper

1 tsp nutmeg, ground

1. Mix together all the ingredients very thoroughly.
2. Season to taste and store in a screw-topped jar in the fridge. Shake vigorously before using. If you make larger quantities, it will keep for at least two weeks if refrigerated.

Respiratory and lymphatic healer

Anne Clark

Avocado Dressing

Makes 1½ cups

1 ripe avocado

1 diced tomato

1 red or green capsicum, diced

3 tbsp minced onion

juice of 1 lemon

2 tbsp oil (optional)

1. Peel and slice avocado and place into a blender and process with the tomato.
2. Add the remaining ingredients while still blending.

Magnesium

Vitamin C

Creamy Nut Dressing

Makes 1–2 cups

1 cup nut meal (almond or hazelnut)

½ cup coconut oil or alternative

½ cup pure water

1 tsp tamari (soy sauce)

1 tsp kelp

1 tsp ground coriander

1. Blend all ingredients.
2. Serve on a vegetable salad. Note if you wish to make a fruit salad dressing, omit the tamari, kelp and coriander and replace with one tablespoon or so of honey.

Kelp – iodine, the metabolism mineral

Lemon Oil Dressing

3 tbsp lemon juice	1. Blend all ingredients together well. Store in refrigerator for up to two weeks. You should have used it all by then!
½ cup coconut oil	
¼ tsp kelp	*Phosphorus, sodium, calcium*
¼ tsp dill, ground	*Vitamin A and C*
1 tbsp honey	

Carrot And Honey Dressing

Makes 1¼ cups

1 cup carrot juice	1. Place all ingredients in a jar with a screw on lid. Shake vigorously until mixed.
2 tbsp minced onion with juices	*Vitamin A*
1 tbsp honey	*Calcium*
1 tsp sesame seeds	

Tomato Herb Dressing

½ clove garlic	1. Process ingredients in an electric blender.
2 tomatoes, quartered	2. Serve on salad of your choice.
2 tbsp sunflower seeds	*Chlorine*
½ tsp each thyme, oregano, rosemary and basil	*Vitamin A and C*

Honey-Peanut Dressing

3 tbsp peanut butter

2 tbsp honey

¼ cup water

3 tbsp lime juice (lemon juice can be used)

1. Process ingredients in an electric blender until smooth. Serve immediately.

High protein

High calorie

Sesame-Soya Dressing

1 cup safflower oil

2 tbsp tamari (soy sauce)

3–4 cloves garlic, chopped

70 g sesame seeds

1. Mix ingredients thoroughly and serve over grated carrots, green salads, or any garden vegetables. Keep stored in the refrigerator.

Rich source of unsaturated lipids

Sweet and Sour Marinade

1 cup pineapple juice, unsweetened

2–3 tbsp Tamari (soy sauce)

1 tbsp lemon juice

garlic, crushed

1. Combine all ingredients in a food processor and blend for one minute. Alternatively, combine in a screw-top jar and shake well. Note: This marinade can be used to enhance the flavour of sprouts and vegetables.

Vitamin C

Digestion aid

Dips and Spreads

If you combine dips and spreads with your salad meals, you will benefit nutritionally and provide an interesting change to your diet.

The following dip and spread recipes are really special to me and are packed with vitamins and minerals. They can all be frozen for later use and keep for up to one week (mushroom dip excluded) in the coldest part of the refrigerator.

Tofu Miso Dip

Makes 1½ cups

375 g tofu

1 tbsp onion juice

3 tsp strong miso

1 tsp ground celery powder

1 tbsp tamari (soy sauce)

1 tbsp shallots, chopped

1. Start by blending the tofu, gradually add onion juice (juice collected from pureed onions) and miso, then continue with the remaining ingredients until the dip is creamy.

2. You may wish to water this dip down to convert it to a salad dressing. This dip is rich in digestible protein.

Protein enriched

The Zinc Dip

Makes 2 cups

- ½ cup pumpkin seeds
- 250 g mushrooms
- 100 g tofu
- 2 tbsp shallots, chopped
- 3 tbsp tahini or peanut paste

1. Soak pumpkin seeds for 8 hours or overnight, then drain.
2. Process the mushrooms with the other ingredients and add the pumpkin seeds. Blend well.
3. Serve with crackers and salad.

Keeps well for two days in refrigerator.

Phosphorus calcium and zinc

Important for low sex drive

Vitamin A helps with stress, fatigue and infection

Cashew Spread

- 150 g cashew nuts
- 1 tbsp shallots, chopped
- 3–4 tbsp tahini (sesame seed paste)
- 1 tbsp water
- 2 tsp miso
- ½ tsp ground nutmeg

1. Process cashew nuts in a food processor until they are finely ground.
2. Gradually add other ingredients and process until all ingredients are combined together well into a creamy spread.
3. Add more water if necessary.

High protein, calcium, magnesium

Important for growth and nerve function

Annie's Classic Peanut, Vegetable and Miso Spread

1 cup shallots, chopped finely

¼ cup chives, chopped

3 cups assorted vegetables (e.g. zucchini, carrot, cabbage, celery), chopped finely

2 tbsp kelp powder

1 tsp coriander seed, ground

1 tsp dark miso

1 clove garlic, crushed

4–5 tbsp peanut paste

water (if necessary)

1. Start by blending all the vegetables with shallots and chives.
2. Add kelp, miso, coriander and garlic, and process well.
3. Add peanut paste. If you would prefer a runny spread, add a little water. This makes several cups, so you may like to freeze small amounts in separate containers for later use.

Alkaline and acid balanced

High in most vitamins and minerals

Radish Spread

Makes 1 cup

85 g radishes, diced

4 tbsp watercress, finely chopped

45 g soy mayonnaise

1. Thoroughly mix the ingredients and refrigerate before serving. Note: Soy mayonnaise is available at health food stores as well as some supermarkets.

Chlorine, silicon and vitamin C

Anne Clark

Almond Vegetable Spread

1 celery stalk, finely chopped

11 mild onion, finely chopped

1 large carrot, finely chopped

350 g almonds, ground

2 tbsp tarragon, finely chopped

2 tbsp caraway seeds, ground

1½ tbsp cumin, ground

1 tbsp curry powder

1½ tsp cayenne pepper

2 tbsp tamari (soy sauce)

1 green capsicum, deseeded and finely chopped

1. Combine the vegetables in a large bowl.
2. Add the remaining ingredients and mix until well blended.
3. This spread should be about the consistency of peanut butter. It is excellent on thick vegetable slices or rounds. It may also be used as a filling for leafy vegetables.

Makes 3 cups

High alkaline

Nearly all vitamin and minerals

Chlorophyll enriched

Sesame-Sunflower Spread

Makes about 4 cups

340 g sesame seeds

340 g sunflower seeds

3 stalks celery, chopped

240 ml sunflower oil

30 g parsley, chopped

1 small onion, coarsely chopped

3 cloves garlic

1 tsp tamari (soy sauce)

1¼ cup lemon juice or more

1. Process the seeds in an electric blender and spoon into a bowl.
2. Process the remaining ingredients until they are liquefied.
3. Combine with the seed mixture and process well.

Essential fatty acids – skin, nails, hair and beauty aid

Vegetable Sandwich Spread

Makes 1 cup

4 tbsp grated cabbage

3 tbsp chopped celery

3 tbsp chopped carrots

3 tbsp chopped green capsicum

2 tbsp soy mayonnaise

1–2 tbsp chopped fresh basil leaves

1. Mix ingredients thoroughly and refrigerate until needed.
2. This spread may also be used as a stuffing for tomatoes. Sprinkle sesame seeds over the top and garnish with basil leaves.

Chlorine cleans the bloodstream

Anne Clark

Vegetarian Pate

Makes 2–3 cups

This is my favourite spread and I really had to do some thinking before I released this prize recipe to the public, but you can't keep everything to yourself, so here it is.

3 celery stalks, chopped finely

3 carrots, chopped finely

½ cup parsley, chopped finely

2 tbsp minced onion

2 tbsp shallots, chopped finely

2 tbsp kelp powder

2 tbsp ground dill

½–1 cup tahini (sesame seed paste)

2 tbsp tamari (soy sauce)

2–3 tbsp lemon juice

1. Start by blending celery, carrots, parsley and onion in your food processor.
2. Add remaining ingredients finishing with tahini and lemon juice.
3. Keep blending all ingredients until you create a thick paste.
4. Scoop mixture out and place it in several plastic containers. Use one straight away and freeze remainder for later use.

Kelp = iodine

Stimulates metabolism

High fibre and low fat

Rich in all vitamins and minerals, especially calcium

In the Raw

Avocado Spread

Makes 1½ cups

1–2 large avocados

1 tomato

¼ tsp minced chilli

1 clove garlic, crushed

sprinkle of black pepper

1. Mash avocados in a medium-sized bowl.
2. Chop tomato finely and add to avocado along with chilli, garlic and black pepper. Mix well. Serve immediately.

Nourishment for nervous system

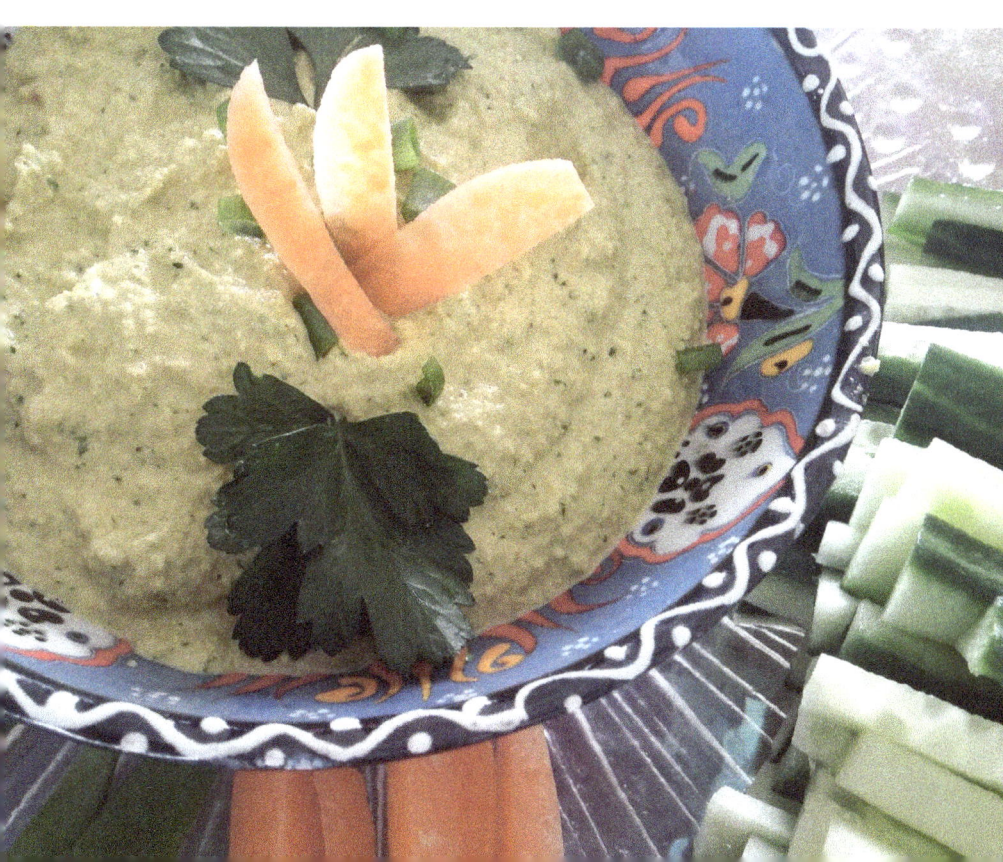

Sweet Spreads And Sauces

Sometimes it's nice to have something to pour over a bowl of fresh fruit or dip fruit pieces into. I hope you'll explore the following suggestions and really impress your friends when you serve your next fruit salad.

Date and Apricot Jam Spread

Makes 3 cups

425 ml warm water

170 g stoned dates

140 g dried apricots

1–2 figs (optional)

1. Process ingredients in a blender until smooth.
2. Serve with fruit.

Note: Any kind of dried fruit can be substituted for the apricots, such as peaches, figs or pears. Soak the fruit in water to soften if desired.

Calcium and phosphorus

Vitamin B1 and B5   Vitamin A   High fibre

Honey-Cinnamon Spread

Makes 1 cup

¼ cup tahini (sesame seed paste)

¾ cup honey

1 tsp ground cinnamon

1. Mix ingredients with a spoon until well blended.
2. Use as a spread for fruit slices or as a sauce over raw fruit puddings.

Calcium

High energy

In the Raw

Apple Sauce

Makes 2½ cups

3 large apples, cored and diced

½ cup apple juice

6 pitted dates or figs

1. Place all ingredients into a blender and process well.
2. Pour mixture into a serving bowl and surround with fruit pieces.

High fibre   Vitamins

Pollution protector

Tropical Fruit Sauce

¼ fresh pineapple, chopped into small chunks

3 sliced bananas

3 soaked figs (keep juice)

1. Place pineapple chunks in blender and liquefy.
2. Add the banana slices and figs and blend until all ingredients become creamy.
3. Serve as sauce or a soup topped with shredded coconut.

Silky Sauce

150 g silken tofu

3 tbsp lemon juice

1 tsp apple juice concentrate

2.5 cm fresh root ginger, peeled and grated

1. Blend the ingredients in a food processor or blender until smooth.

Vitamin A & C for colds and infections

Anne Clark

Almond Cream

Makes 1 cup

Serve this cream over raspberries, blackberries or strawberries. It really is a special treat and very helpful for people who suffer from fatigue or skin problems and if you are feeling out of sorts.

125 g almonds

75 ml apple juice

1. Put the almonds in a blender or food processor with the apple juice, and blend or process until creamy.
2. Spoon the cream over fruit.

High magnesium

Strong bones and teeth

Memory

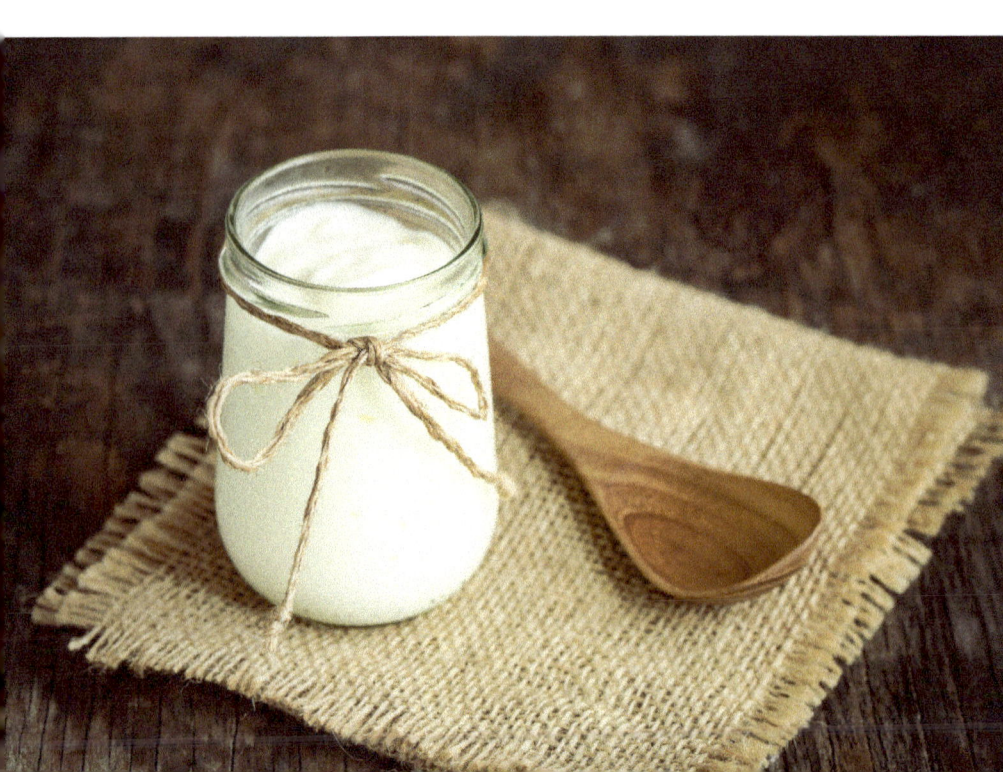

Bread

I am frequently asked about the benefit of bread:

"Do we need it?"

"Is it healthy?"

"Where does it fit in with raw food?"

Hmm...that is a tricky one and can only be answered in two parts.

Bread is usually made from flour which has been processed from the grain. Now, unless you are growing your own wheat and then grinding the grain on stone and preparing your bread immediately, you will never get the real nutritional benefit from wheat, rye or any other grain bread. Bread is usually cooked and, when combined with avocado and sprouts, can be a complete meal. However, avocado and sprouts together can also be a balanced combination and you could easily survive without the bread which I consider a luxury anyway. If your diet consists of mainly 75% raw foods (fresh fruits and vegetables), a piece of bread here and there will do no harm. It is only when your concentrated foods (grains, seeds, nuts and animal products) far exceed your fresh foods that you should seriously consider cutting back on bread.

For the benefit of all those people who have asked me for suitable recipes for bread, I think the following ideas will help you. Breadmaking is usually quite lengthy and precise with temperature being one important aspect. The first recipe relieves these worries as it is as close to raw as you will find and filled with valuable nutrients.

Anne Clark

Sprouted Mung Bean Bread

- 2½–3 cups sprouted mung beans
- 2–3 tbsp rolled oats (more if necessary)
- 2–3 tbsp rice bran (to make firmer)
- 1–2 tbsp wheatgerm

1. Place mung beans in a food processor and process completely.
2. Add rolled oats gradually while machine is still processing.
3. Remove from the food processor and add the rice bran and wheatgerm. Mix well.
4. Pat as flat as possible into two greased trays.
5. Place out in the sun for half the day or dry out in a warm oven (temperature no higher than 120ºC) for 30–45 minutes.
6. Allow to cool. Slice into sections and enjoy with dips and spreads of your choice.

Low fat   High B vitamins

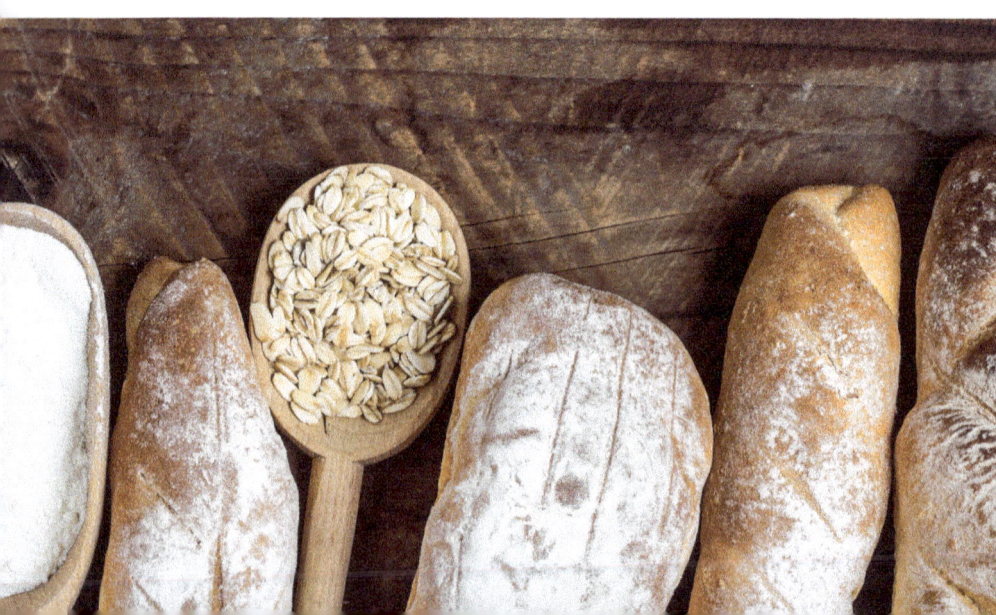

Unyeasted Bread

Makes 1 loaf

2 cups wholemeal flour

2 cups whole rye (sprouted and ground slightly in blender)

½ tsp caraway seeds

2 cups water

2 tbsp honey

1. Mix flour, ground rye and caraway seeds together. Add water mixed with honey gradually.
2. Knead for ten minutes.
3. Place in an oiled bread pan and cover with a damp cloth.
4. Let rise for several hours or overnight in a warm place.
5. Bake for 2–3 hours in a 180°C oven.
6. Note: For a moister loaf up to one tablespoon of oil can be added for each cup of flour.

B-complex vitamins & vitamin E

Carob Bread

Makes 1 loaf

2 cups pitted dates, chopped

1 cup raisins, chopped

½ cup carob powder

water (optional)

1. Process dates, raisins and carob powder in a food processor.
2. Add more carob powder if necessary and a little water (optional). The dough should be sufficiently stiff to roll out.
3. Roll out dough and cut into wafers, bite size or larger.
4. Expose to the sunshine for several hours to dry slightly.

High fibre   Gentle laxative

Anne Clark

Falafel Flat Bread

Makes 6–8

- 15 g fresh yeast
- 300 ml warm water
- 1 tsp honey
- 250 g unbleached flour or 1 tsp dried yeast
- 1 tsp olive oil
- 250 g wholemeal flour
- 1 tsp tamari (soy sauce)

1. Dissolve yeast in a small amount of the warm water. Add honey and leave to froth in a warm place.

2. Sift both flours into a bowl. Make a well in the centre and pour in the yeast mix.

3. Knead well, adding enough of the remaining water to make a firm but not hard dough. Knead well on a floured board for about 15 minutes until the dough is smooth and no longer sticks to your fingers. Knead in one or two tablespoons of oil for a softer bread.

4. Sprinkle a board with oil and roll the ball of dough round to grease it all over and prevent the surface from becoming dry and crusty. Cover with a damp cloth and leave in a warm place for two hours, until nearly doubled in size.

5. Punch dough down and knead again for a few minutes.

6. Take a potato-sized lump and roll out with a floured rolling pin as thin as possible (less than 1 cm thick so that they puff up more and leave a better pouch) approximately 14cm diameter.

7. Dust each round with flour and lay on a cloth sprinkled with flour. Cover with another lightly floured cloth and allow to rise again in a warm place. You may like to brush dough with some tamari.

8. Preheat oven to 200°C and heat oiled baking sheets.

9. When bread has risen, arrange on baking sheets and bake for 6–10 minutes.

10. Remove from baking sheets. Bread should be soft and white with a

pouch inside. If not using immediately, place in a sealed plastic bag so they stay soft.

Whole wheat flour is high in B vitamins.

There is some nutritional loss due to heat (cooking)

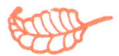

Annie's Dip Biscuits

These dip biscuits are classed as part of my bread foods. I have already mentioned that rice cakes (available from health food shops and supermarkets) are also part of my diet and very occasionally I like to incorporate some of these biscuits into my diet as well. They are really something, and I know you and your friends will love them.

3 cups wholemeal flour	1. Mix the flour with herbs, cumin and coriander.
2 tbsp mixed dried herbs	2. Add the mayonnaise, oil, soy sauce, coriander and enough water to form a dough. Be careful not to add too much water.
1 tsp cumin	
2 tbsp soy sauce	3. Knead on a floured board. Roll out flat and cut into shapes.
2 tbsp soy mayonnaise or peanut butter	
1–2 tbsp olive oil	4. Place shapes on greased trays and bake for 15 minutes in a 180°C oven.
1 tsp coriander or alternative	
water	

The healthy snack biscuit

B vitamins

Flat Crackers

These crackers can be plain or add a handful of either sesame seeds, poppy seeds, linseeds (flax seeds), aniseeds, caraway seeds or fennel seeds to each portion to make a variety batch of crackers.

Ingredients	Method
1 cup rye flour	1. Combine dry ingredients in a bowl.
1 cup soy flour	2. Boil water and add oil and honey.
1½ cup wholemeal flour	3. Combine well, pour and stir into flour. Use enough water to make a soft pliable dough (not sticky).
1 cup oatmeal	4. Knead for ten minutes.
⅓–½ cup olive oil	5. Either divide into 12 equal portions and roll lightly outwards from the centre until paper thin or use a cookie sheet and cut into equal sizes.
1½ cup boiling water	
1 tbsp honey	
	6. Bake in oven at 200°C for 15–20 minutes, or until thoroughly dried and slightly browned.

High protein

High energy

In the Raw

Wheat And Rye Biscuits

Makes 12 x 10cm biscuits

- 115 g wheat sprouts
- 115 g rye sprouts
- 2 tsp crushed caraway seeds
- 1 small onion, chopped finely
- 1 tbsp kelp powder
- 1 tbsp fresh parsley, chopped finely

1. Mix ingredients and put through a food processor. The mixture should be sticky, but firm.
2. Roll into 5cm balls, then press flat.
3. Place the flattened balls between two sheets of greaseproof paper and roll out to a thickness of approximately 3cm. The thinner they are rolled, the quicker they will dry and the crisper they will be.
4. Place the biscuits on wire mesh in the sunshine or in a food dryer.

Athlete's training fuel

Vitamin & mineral enriched

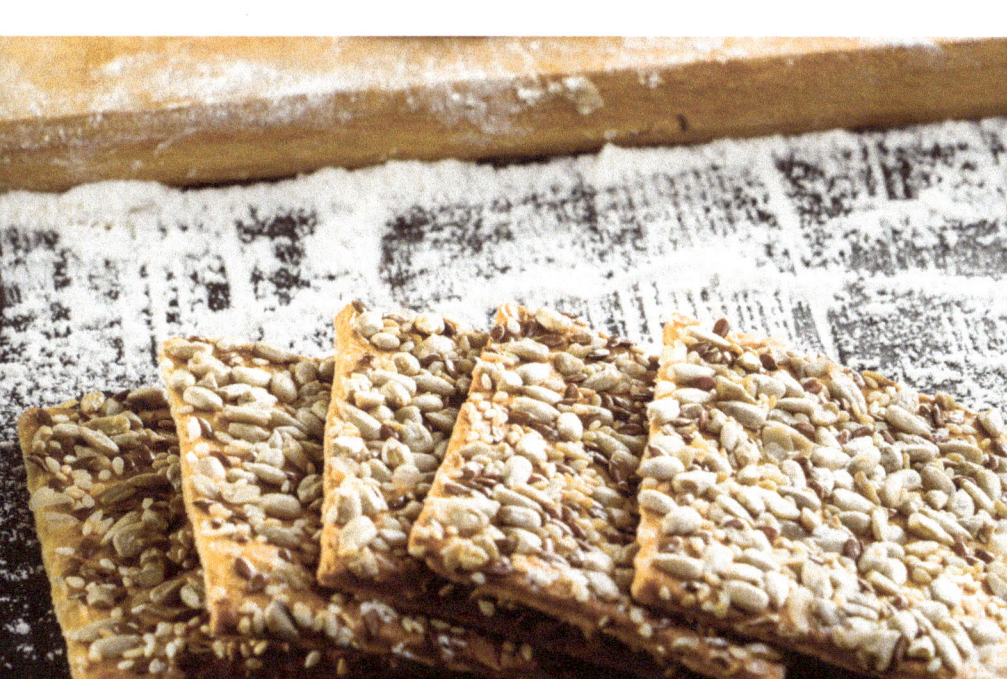

Anne Clark

Celebration Bread

Makes approx. 30

This bread takes time and is a bit fiddly but the result is worth the effort. Not everyone will like them, but I think they are magnificent. The recipe calls for sprouted wheat and aduki bean sprouts, which can be substituted with mung bean sprouts if you wish. Be sure to use plenty of oatmeal to help form your flat bread shapes.

2½ cups sprouted organic wheat

1½ cups aduki bean sprouts

½ cup sesame seeds

1 cup oatmeal

1 tsp tamari (soy sauce)

extra oatmeal for rolling out bread

1. Begin by blending the sprouts with sesame seeds, tamari and oatmeal. Add more oatmeal if you think it is necessary.

2. Form small balls and pat out as flat as you can (approx. 7–8cm diameter). Use the extra oatmeal to prevent sticking.

3. Place each round on a wire rack with a tray underneath and place out in the warm sun for 6–7 hours. Alternatively, you may wish to dry them out in the oven on a very low heat.

4. When firm, place in a sealed container and store in the refrigerator.

Enzymes are sensitive to heat

Sprouts are living food!

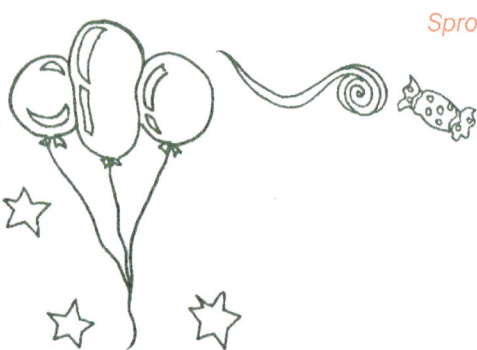

Sesame Tofu Crackers

Makes 50 crackers

3 cups unbleached white flour or whole wheat flour

3 tbsp sesame seeds

1 tsp baking powder

125 g tofu

½ cup olive oil

¼ cup water

1. Mix dry ingredients together in a bowl.
2. In a blender, blend tofu, olive oil and water together until smooth and creamy:
3. Make a well in the middle of the dry ingredients and pour in the blended mix. Mix well. Add up to ¼ cup of water if necessary to make a soft dough.
4. Roll out on a lightly floured board as thin as possible and cut diagonally into strips.
5. Bake for 12–15 minutes at 200°C or until golden brown. Watch them carefully so they don't burn.
6. These will keep well if stored in an airtight container.

Good supply of B vitamins, iron, phosphorus, sodium, potassium and fat-soluble vitamin E

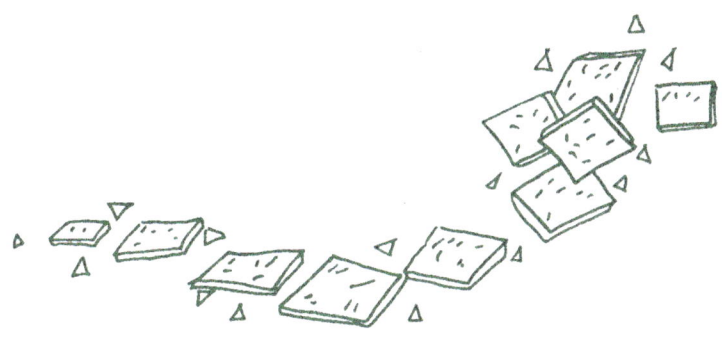

Anne Clark

Main Dishes

Raw foods in your life doesn't have to mean depressing mounds of unlikely plant life that you are expected to chomp your way through as though you were grazing in a paddock. For most of you the following recipes will be a new experience.

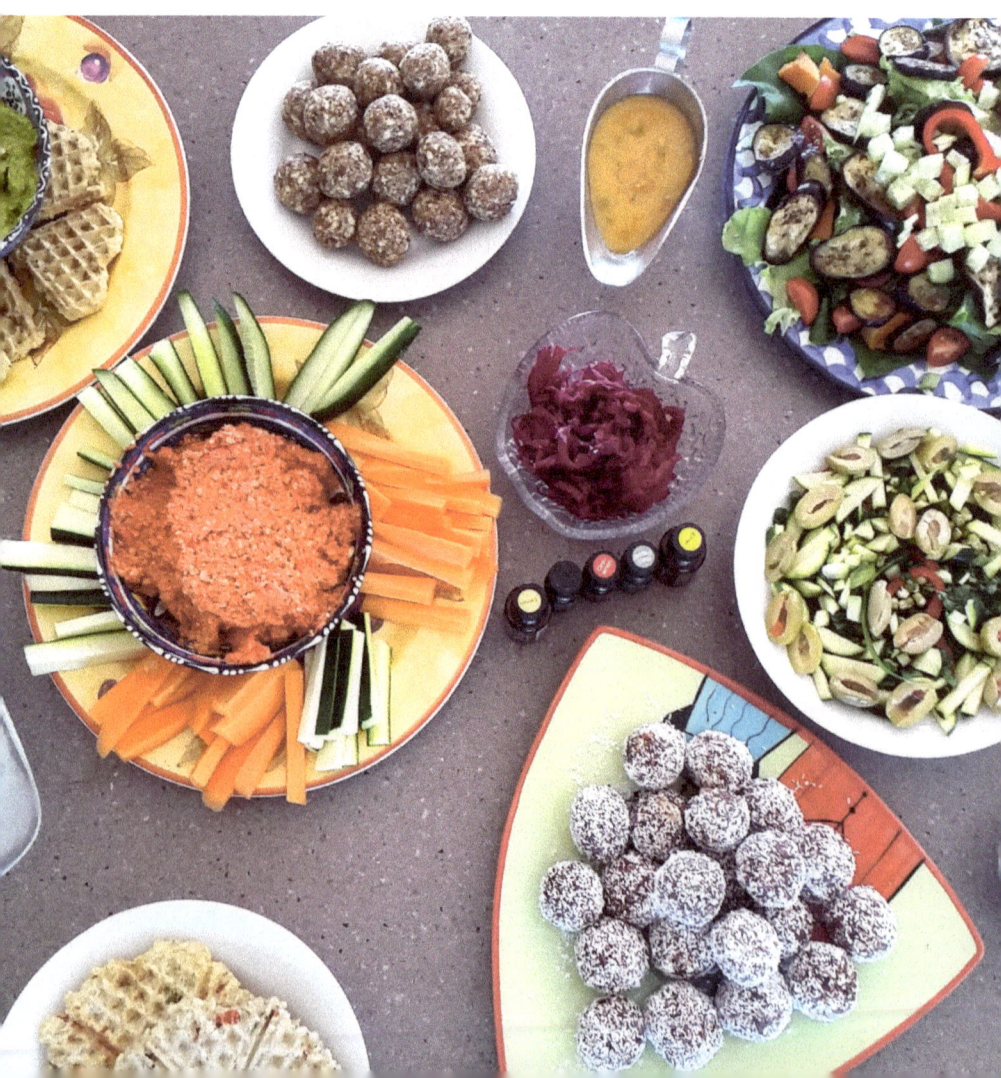

The Sprout Roll

Serves 6–8

The sprout roll is just one of those incredible combinations that not only satisfies a hungry person but contributes to a glowing skin and happy light feeling afterwards. To me that is worth so much because I look at my food as the booster to help me carry out my thinking, exercise and creativity. Try the sprout roll first and serve it with any of my lovely salads.

Ingredients	Method
115 g alfalfa sprouts	1. Mix together the sprouts, onion and garlic.
30 g soya beansprouts	2. Add the lemon juice, kelp powder and soy sauce.
30 g lentil sprouts	3. Place a portion of the sprout mixture in the centre of a lettuce leaf and repeat the procedure with the remaining lettuce leaves.
30 g wheat sprouts	
4 tbsp onion, finely chopped	
1 clove garlic, finely chopped	4. Top with avocado and tomato slices.
juice of 1 lemon	5. Roll up and secure with a toothpick if necessary.
½ tsp kelp powder	
1 tsp tamari (soy sauce)	
6–8 lettuce leaves	
1 avocado, sliced	
1 tomato, sliced	

Complete vitamin & minerals

All essential amino acids

Balanced in fats, proteins & carbohydrates

Anne Clark

Avocado & Almond Supreme

Serves 6

- 4 ripe avocados, peeled, halved and stoned
- juice of 2 lemons
- 1 tsp basil leaves
- ½ tsp sage
- pinch of black pepper
- 455 g celery, finely chopped
- 115 g carrots, grated
- 85 g cabbage, finely chopped
- 4 tbsp diced onions
- 4 tbsp chopped parsley
- sprouts of salad to serve
- ½ cup ground almonds

1. Mash the avocados with the lemon juice, then blend in basil, sage and pepper.
2. Combine with the celery, carrots, cabbage, onions and parsley.
3. Form into a round loaf and place on a bed of sprouts or salad. Top with ground almonds.

Calcium

Vitamin A & C

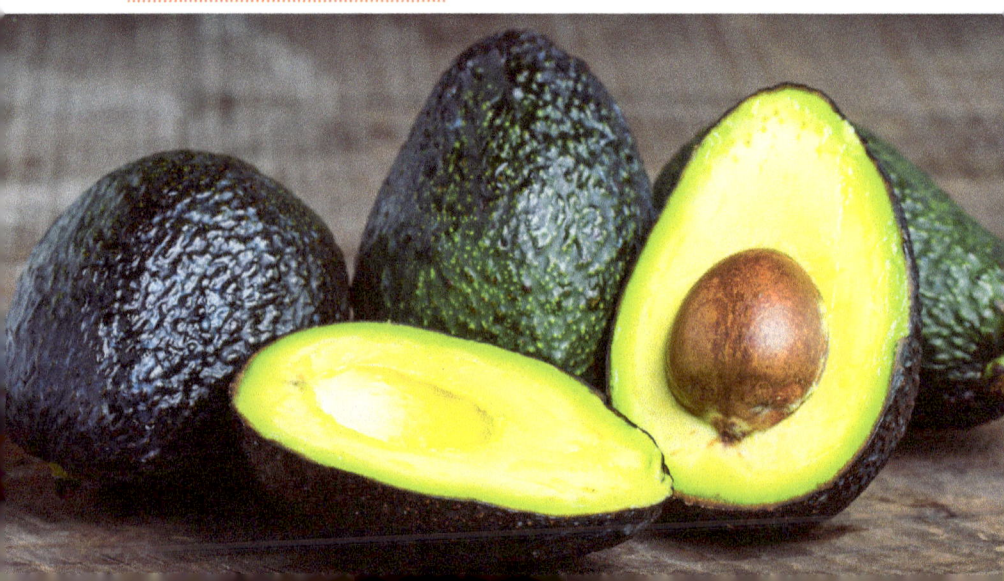

Hazelnut Loaf

1 cup ground hazelnuts

125 g carrots, grated

1 onion, chopped finely

½ cup oats

1 tsp fresh sage, chopped

1 tsp fresh thyme, chopped

1 tsp French mustard

1 tsp sunflower oil

50 ml vegetable stock or water

1. Blend hazelnuts with carrots, onion, oats, herbs, mustard and oil until thoroughly combined.
2. Gradually add the water or vegetable stock and blend until the mixture is just wet enough to hold together. It will firm up when left. Season to taste.
3. Press into a loaf tin lined with greaseproof paper.
4. Leave to stand for one hour, then turn out and place on a plate lined with lettuce leaves. Serve with my traditional mayonnaise.

Vitamin B5 & B6

Vitamin A

Protein enriched

Anne Clark

Patties

Makes 12

These patties are fairly simple to make and there is minimum preparation involved if you use cooked rice but do try the sprouted wheat version as well.

1 cup brown rice (cooked) or sprouted wheat

¼ cup diced capsicum

2 tbsp lemon juice

2 stalks of celery, chopped

1 tbsp honey (optional)

¼ cup grated carrot

1 ripe avocado, mashed

fresh herbs, chopped

1. Mix ingredients together well.
2. Form into pattie shapes.
3. Roll in ground peanuts, chill and serve.

B-complex vitamins

Energy & stress relief

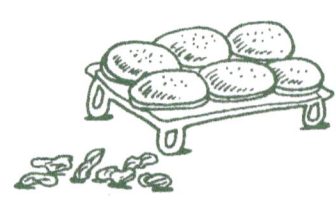

Vegetable Nut Loaf

1 cup grated carrots

1 cup chopped celery

1 cup chopped broccoli

½ cup shallots, chopped

½ cup sunflower seeds

½ cup assorted nuts, ground

1 cup boiling water

1 tbsp agar

1 tbsp lemon juice

1 tsp honey

1. Mix together the carrot, celery, broccoli, shallots, sunflower seeds and nuts in a medium-sized bowl. Set aside.
2. Mix together the boiling water, agar, lemon juice and honey until the agar dissolves. Add to the vegetable and nut mix and mix well.
3. Chill until set. Serve with lettuce and grated raw beetroot.

Vitamin A, C & E

Essential fatty acids

Celery Nut Loaf

2 cups celery, finely grated or ground

3 tbsp minced parsley

1 cup ground almonds

juice of 1 small lemon

1 mashed avocado

½ tsp thyme

3 tbsp minced onion

2 tbsp mayonnaise

1. Mix all ingredients together and pack into a loaf pan.
2. Chill for several hours before serving. Serve with some sort of nut sauce, dip or pate.

Calcium

Magnesium

Potassium

Sodium

Anne Clark

Squash with Basil and Sesame

Serves 2

This recipe is also presented in my book Two Weeks to Better Health where it is cooked, however I discovered just how wonderful it tastes raw also.

6 green or yellow squash

1 tbsp sesame seeds

1 tbsp olive oil

1 small onion (approx. ¼ cup when chopped finely)

1 tbsp fresh basil, chopped finely

1 tbsp tahini (sesame seed paste)

1 tsp tamari (soy sauce)

1 tsp honey

1 tsp white miso (optional)

extra sesame seeds if needed

1. Trim a slice from the base of each squash so they sit flat. Scoop a shallow round from the top of each squash. Take the pieces of squash cut from the base and top of each squash and combine with the remaining ingredients.

2. Place all ingredients into a food processor (except the squash that will be stuffed). Blend or process the filling until the mixture resembles a puree.

3. Spoon the mixture into the prepared squash and serve with a sprinkle of sesame seeds. Serve immediately as a main meal with salad or as an entree with other stuffed vegetables.

Vitamin A

Calcium

Great for slimmers

Savoury Balls

Makes 24

Savoury balls can be as complicated or as simple as you like, but I like to keep them simple. Start with the basic recipe presented here and add on ingredients that suit you and your particular situation (i.e. what is available and fresh). Using the seeds will ensure that you get adequate protein and essential minerals like calcium and zinc.

½ cup pumpkin seeds

½ cup sunflower seeds

½ cup sesame seeds

1–2 tbsp minced onion

1 tsp tamari (soy sauce)

1 cup grated carrot or pumpkin

fresh parsley, chopped finely

1 tsp lemon juice

1. Start by processing the seeds in your food processor until they resemble fine breadcrumbs.

2. Add onion, grated vegetables and soy sauce. Finish with parsley and lemon juice.

3. Scoop the mixture out and store in the refrigerator for 24 hours to make the mixture easier to shape (and it also improves the flavour!).

4. Shape the mixture into small balls then roll in sesame seeds. Serve on a bed of lettuce and enjoy with salad. Once the savoury balls are made they will only keep for 2–3 days in the refrigerator.

Protein

Calcium & iron

Pea Patties

Makes 12

- 2 cups fresh peas
- ½ cup sunflower seeds
- 2 cups diced, raw carrots
- ½ cup shallots, chopped finely
- 2 tsp kelp powder
- pinch of oregano

1. Process the peas, carrots, shallots and sunflower seeds in your food processor.
2. Mix in the kelp and oregano.
3. Form into patties. Top with mayonnaise or one of my dips.

Potassium & Vitamin A

Great for slimmers

Nut Loaf

- 1 cup carrots
- 1 cup tomatoes or cucumber, chopped finely
- ½ cup chopped parsley
- ½ cup capsicum, chopped finely
- 1 clove garlic
- 2 tbsp oil
- ground nuts
- sprinkle of dill or sage

1. Place all ingredients in a food processor.
2. Process well and pack into a loaf pan to serve or make as a sandwich filling. Can be served as a pate or dip by adding tahini. Serve immediately.

Vitamin A & C

Athlete's fuel

Vegetable Loaf

- 8 carrots
- ½ bunch of celery
- 1 capsicum
- 1 bunch of shallots
- 1 cup ground sunflower seeds
- ½ cup whole sunflower seeds
- ½ cup tahini (sesame seed paste)
- vegetable seasoning to taste
- caraway seeds, ground
- 1 tbsp oregano
- 1 tbsp cumin
- 1 tbsp parsley

1. Juice the carrots. Serve the juice. Put the pulp in a large bowl.
2. Mince the celery, capsicum and shallots finely, and add to the carrot pulp.
3. Mix in the remaining ingredients and blend all ingredients together well by hand.
4. Put the mixture into a baking dish or baking pan and incubate in the sun for 6–8 hours (the incubation makes a crust). Serve as a main course with salad and dips.

Complete protein

High fibre

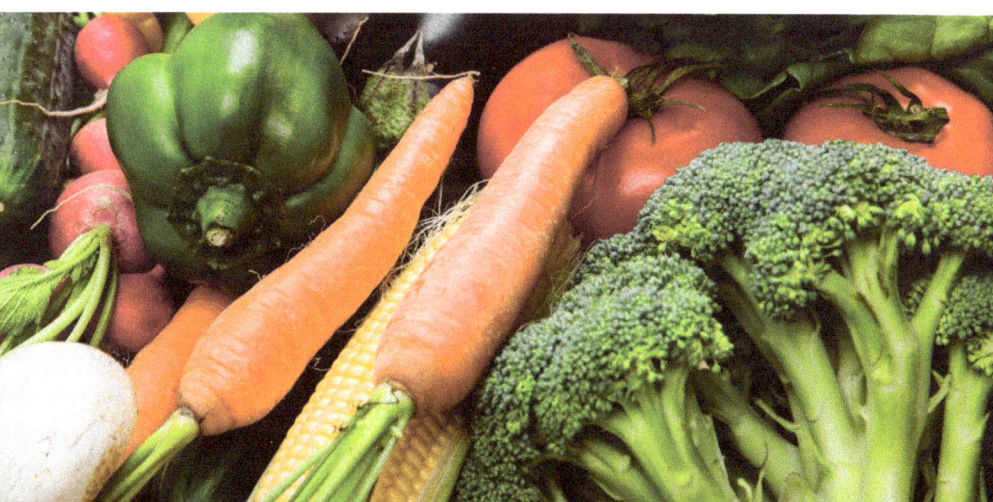

Sweet Treats and Desserts

Everyone likes a treat and nearly everyone I know has had an addiction to something sweet. If it isn't chocolate, it's something else. Now I need to explain something very important here in order for you to respect the direction that I'm coming from:

It is not necessary to eat desserts! They should not be part of your diet!

With all the bad press surrounding consumption of sugar, you may be wondering why I include a section on sweet treats and desserts in this book. Some of the most exciting taste sensations come from blending dried fruits and nuts together and forming little balls or bases for fruit pies and desserts which are healthy. Now if you are eating right with a balance of raw vegetables, sprouts, seeds, nuts and fruits, then the addition of a few treats will not hurt, but I stress that you must not sustain yourself on sweet treats alone. That is totally out of balance and will only contribute to your downfall, not only in health but in mental reasoning as well. Too many sweet foods in your diet will cause a chemical imbalance which can lead to all sorts of problems. Just take my word for it. So make up some of these treats, but do not go crazy.

In honour of my loyal customers and clients who have asked for recipes for the raw food treats that showed up on my market stall at Kuranda Market or Noosa Harbour or were offered when friends came to visit, I've dedicated this part of my book to them. I feel they deserve to share the joy of such healthy and yummy treats and when I come to visit maybe I'll get to try some of their new creations...maybe!

In the Raw

Not all my secrets will I share,
But just a few to show I care.
Treats in life are wants not needs,
Better one thinks and reads!

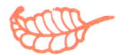

Fruit Pie Crust No.1

You can make so many different fruit pies and the pie crust can make or break the whole taste of your pie. This crust is very filling and rich in protein. If you are watching your weight, just a little piece won't hurt, but better not to make it at all if you can't control yourself. This recipe makes enough for one average pie shell.

1 cup almonds

½ cup hazelnuts

½ cup sunflower seeds

2 tbsp peanut paste

1 tsp cinnamon, ground

1–2 tbsp water

1. Process nuts and seeds in your food processor.
2. Add peanut paste, cinnamon and water, and process until the mixture resembles a tough dough.
3. Press into a pie shell which has been lightly greased with oil.
4. Refrigerate while preparing filling. Crust can be frozen for up to two months before use.

Useful as a raw cookie mix

High calorie

High protein

Anne Clark

Fruit Pie Crust No.2

¼ cup almonds

2 cups rolled oats

¼ cup raisins, chopped

¼ cup lime, lemon, orange or pineapple juice

1 tsp vanilla essence

water (if necessary)

1. Begin by processing the almonds until finely ground.
2. Add rolled oats and process.
3. Add raisins, citrus juice of your choice and vanilla essence. Only use water if the mixture appears too crumbly and dry.
4. Process all ingredients well. The mixture should resemble a tough dough.
5. Press mixture into prepared pie shell (greased with a little oil).
6. Refrigerate while preparing filling.

Note: This mixture can be transformed into raw cookies as well. Simply roll mixture into little balls the size of a walnut and press flat. Stud each piece with an almond and chill.

Calcium and high fibre

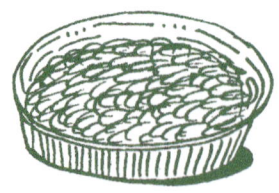

Banana-Date Pie

This following recipe makes enough to fill a 23cm pie shell.

3 bananas, sliced and frozen

4 stoned dates

1 tsp ground cinnamon

½ cup apple juice (approx.)

1 chilled piecrust

sprinkle of nuts

1. Combine the bananas and dates in a blender, adding just enough apple juice to process until creamy.
2. Pour into the piecrust and sprinkle cinnamon and nuts over the top.
3. Chill and serve.

Calcium, potassium & magnesium

Relieves constipation

Banana Truffles

Makes 12

2 ripe bananas, mashed

1–2 tbsp tahini

2 cups pitted dates, chopped

½ cup raisins, chopped

½ cup pecan nuts, chopped

2 cups desiccated coconut

1. Mix together banana, tahini, dates, raisins, nuts and one cup coconut.
2. Form into balls about the size of a walnut.
3. Roll the balls in the remaining coconut and chill in the refrigerator. Keeps well for up to a week.

Biotin, calcium & iron

Ideal for young children

Anne Clark

Main Attraction Salad

Serves 4

2 ripe mangoes

1 kiwi fruit, peeled and thinly sliced into 8 slices

12 large strawberries

½ cup passionfruit pulp

1. Cut the mangoes in half with a serrated knife. Slip the knife under the flat pit and remove four halves. Allow one half mango per serve. Score each half into 3cm cubes, making sure you do not cut the skin. Fold each half mango back to fan out the cubes and place slightly off-centre on your serving plate.

2. Slice three strawberries and place overlapping slices on two sides of the mango.

3. Then place two slices of kiwi on the third side.

4. Spoon some passionfruit pulp on the empty side of the plate and the remainder over the fruits. Repeat for other serves.

5. Chill and serve.

Skin & beauty aid

Vitamin C enriched

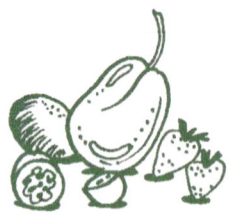

Dates with Orange

Serves 6

- 6 navel oranges
- 12 fresh dates
- ¼ cup orange juice
- cinnamon
- ¼ cup sliced almonds

1. Remove peel from one orange, cut into needle thin julienne strips for garnish and set aside. Remove pith and membrane and slice each orange horizontally into thin slices with a serrated bread knife. Arrange the orange slices in an overlapping circle on individual serving plates.

2. Allow two dates for each serve. Split each date vertically and remove the pits. Mince one date per serving and scatter over the orange slices. Arrange the two halves of the other date in the centre of the orange slices.

3. Spoon over the orange juice, then sprinkle with cinnamon and scatter one teaspoon sliced of almonds and julienned peel over each plate.

4. Cover, chill and serve.

Vitamin A & C

Great for high energy people

Anne Clark

Hollywood Bananas

Serves 4

½ cup pureed mango

½ cup pureed blueberries

2–3 bananas, peeled and sliced diagonally

lemon juice

2 starfruit (carambola), cut thinly

green leaves for garnish

a few strawberries for garnish

a few grapes for garnish

1. Spoon two tablespoons of the mango puree on one half of a dinner plate.
2. Spoon two tablespoons of blueberry puree on the other half of the plate.
3. Place 8–9 overlapping slices of banana in rows on one side of the plate where the two sauces meet.
4. Squeeze lemon juice over the banana.
5. Lay slices of starfruit in the blueberry puree and decorate with strawberries and grapes.
6. Repeat procedure for each serving.

Vitamin A, B-complex & C

Cleansing food

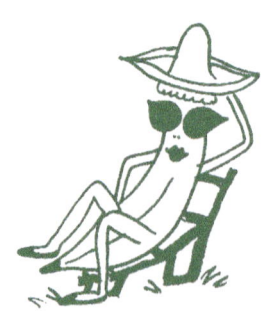

Apple & Fig Slice

Makes 12 slices

This slice makes a wonderful afternoon snack. It is rich in iron and fibre, so not only is it a great pick-me-up, it will keep you regular as well. This mixture makes enough for one average size lamington tray (approx. 30cm x 20cm).

16 soaked figs (reserve soaking juice)

2 cups almonds in their skins

1 cup dried apples, chopped finely

2 tbsp fig nectar

1 tsp vanilla essence

1 tbsp honey (optional)

1. Drain the soaked figs thoroughly. Reserve the juice (use some for the recipe).

2. Add soaked figs to remaining ingredients and place all into a food processor and process until well combined.

3. Spread into a well-greased lamington tray and chill. Slice and wrap in individual slices.

High fibre helps concentration

Carob Fudge

Makes 10 slices

1¼ cups carob powder

⅓ cup warm water

5 tbsp honey

2 tsp vanilla essence

2 tbsp tahini

1½ cups pecan or walnuts, chopped finely

1. Mix carob powder with warm water to make a smooth paste.
2. Heat the honey, vanilla and tahini, then add to the carob mixture, together with the nuts.
3. Mix well together, pour into a lightly greased square tin and refrigerate. Cut into squares before set. Store in the refrigerator.

Rich in B vitamins   Provides energy

Fruit & Carob Fudge

Makes 12 slices

This is a richer version of carob fudge and in my opinion even better!

½ cup honey

½ cup peanut butter

⅓ cup carob powder

¼ cup soy milk powder

2 cups ground mixed nuts or seeds

½ cup sultanas, chopped finely

½ cup coconut

1. Heat the honey and add peanut butter, then add all other ingredients.
2. Spoon into an oiled 20cm square dish and refrigerate until firm. Cut into squares or slices and store in the refrigerator.

Protein enriched

Eat in moderation

In the Raw

Fruit & Seed Bar

Makes 12 slices

¼ cup sunflower seeds

2 tbsp sesame seeds

1 cup chopped raisins

1 cup sultanas, chopped

½ cup dried apples, chopped

juice of ½ orange (3 tbsp approx.)

1. Place sunflower seeds and sesame seeds in a food processor first. Process until well ground.
2. Gradually add the remaining ingredients and process until you are happy with the consistency.
3. Scoop the mixture out of the processor and press into a wetted baking tray and sprinkle with more sesame seeds.
4. Chill, slice and wrap. Can also be used as a base for a fruit pie.

Calcium & magnesium

Great for students

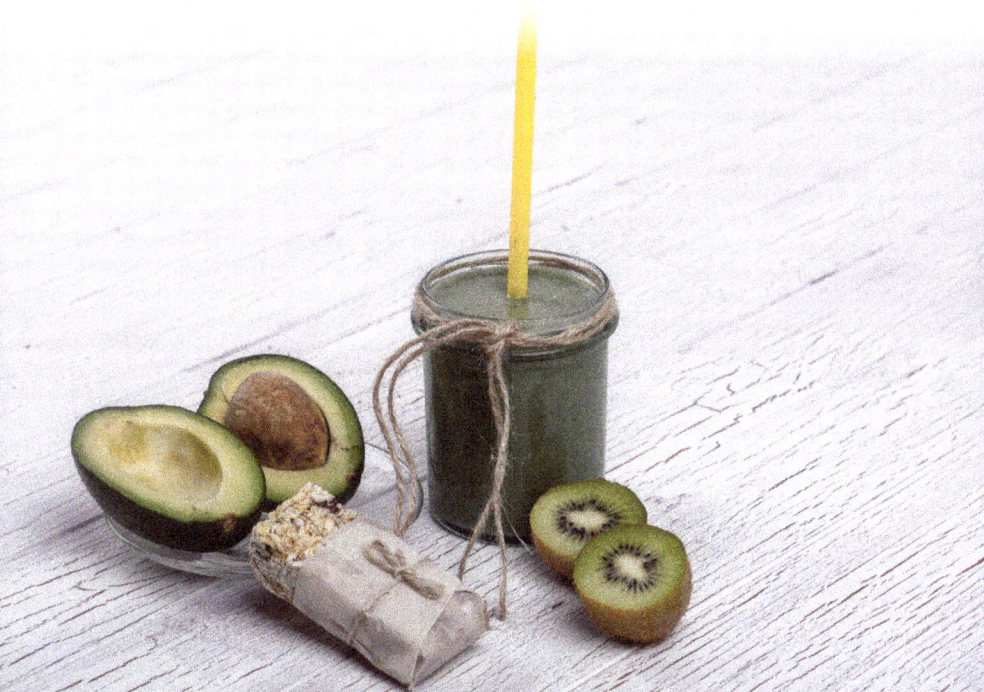

Anne Clark

Hazelnut Rough

Makes 12 slices

- 2 cups oatmeal
- 2 cups ground hazelnuts
- 1 cup sesame seeds
- 1 cup coconut
- ½ cup honey
- ½ cup carob powder
- 1 tbsp caro (coffee alternative)
- 1 tsp vanilla essence
- water

1. Combine all ingredients, adding enough water to bind (not too much).
2. Press into a greased lamington tray.
3. Chill, slice and wrap into bars. Keeps very well in the refrigerator.

Vitamin A & calcium

High fibre

Great winter treat

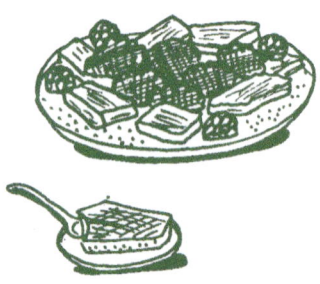

Peanut Halva

Makes 12

This is one of my most popular slices. I sold this delight from my Kuranda Market stall and people always came back to tell me how much they liked it. As it is very high in calories, I suggest you eat it in moderation and never at the end of the night or before you retire as it will take a while to digest.

1 cup sunflower seeds

1 cup pumpkin seeds

1 cup peanuts

½ cup peanut paste

½ cup honey

1 tsp vanilla essence

1. Start by processing the seeds in your food processor.
2. Add the nuts and process until mixture is well ground.
3. Add honey and peanut paste mixed with vanilla essence. Process to combine.
4. Press mixture into a greased lamington tray.
5. Chill, slice and wrap.

Protein enriched

Essential fatty acids

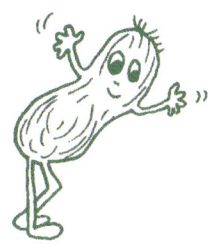

Pecan Cacao Pie

1 cup pecan nuts

½ cup cacao powder

½ cup softened or melted coconut oil

½ cup maple syrup or honey

1 tsp vanilla essence

2 tbsp almond meal or dōTERRA V Shake

1 pinch sea salt

1 drop dōTERRA essential oil of Cinnamon Bark

½ cup desiccated coconut

½ cup extra pecans for decoration

1. Blend all ingredients in food processor, except for extra pecans for decoration.
2. Line a small square or round glass dish with baking paper.
3. Scoop mixture into the dish.
4. Top and press with extra pecans.
5. Place creation into the freezer and chill for at least one hour.

High protein

Essential fatty acids

Brain food

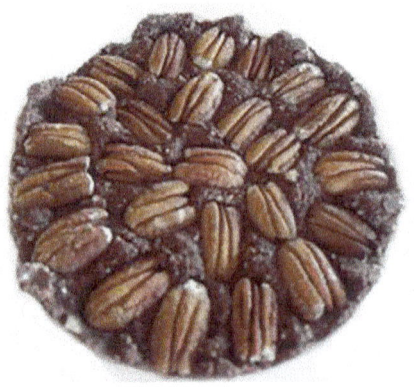

In the Raw

Fruit & Nut Bar

Makes 12 bars

¾ cups chopped peanuts or almonds

1½ cups peaches, chopped finely

2 cups raisins, chopped finely

juice of ½ orange (approx. 3 tbsp)

extra chopped peanuts

1. In a food processor, grind together all the dried fruits and nuts. Process until they hold together.
2. Add orange juice to moisten.
3. Press mixture into a greased lamington tray. Sprinkle nuts over the top.
4. Chill, slice and wrap. Will keep for up to 1 month in the refrigerator.

High in Vitamin A

Potassium & phosphorus

Weight builder's slice

Apricot Coconut Bars

Makes 10 slices

1 cup dried apricots, chopped

2 cups grated coconut

2 tbsp honey

½ cup pecans, chopped

2 tbsp almond nut cream, thick

1. Soak apricots till soft. Drain well.
2. Add coconut, honey, pecans and almond cream. Mix well.
3. Press into a wetted lamington tray.
4. Refrigerate for 2–3 hours then serve sliced into bar shapes.

Vitamin A enriched

Calcium & magnesium

Anne Clark

Fruit Kababs

Use any tropical fruit in season. Cut into bite-sized pieces. Place on skewers. Serve on a large platter for a luncheon dessert or for the whole luncheon itself.

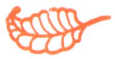

Fruit Bites

Makes 20

These little delicacies can be served after dinner or lunch and also make an ideal afternoon snack. We eat them on bushwalks and appreciate the energy boost they give in return. They will keep for several months in the fridge but our fruit bites are never around long enough to worry.

1 tbsp honey

1 cup almonds

1 cup mixed dried fruit (such as dates and apricots)

¼ cup orange juice or apple juice (optional)

coconut or sesame seeds for decoration

1. Place nuts in a food processor and chop thoroughly.
2. Add dried fruit and continue to process as you add the honey and enough fruit juice to make the mixture bind.
3. Remove the mixture from the processor and roll into balls with coconut.
4. Chill in the fridge and serve when suitable.

Protein and fibre

In the Raw

Raw Carob Brownies

Makes 16

- 1–2 cups oatmeal
- ½ cup carob powder
- ¼ cup sesame seeds
- ¼ cup sunflower seeds
- ½ cup honey
- 2 cups mixed nuts
- 1 tsp vanilla essence
- water

1. Grind nuts well in a food processor.
2. Combine all the ingredients in a medium-sized bowl adding water if necessary to help mixture to bind. Be careful not to add too much water.
3. Press mixture into a lamington tray. Chill and cut into bars or squares to serve.

Note: You can freeze the slices individually and pack them with the children's lunches as they can survive out of the fridge for a few days.

Essential fatty acids

Potassium & phosphorus

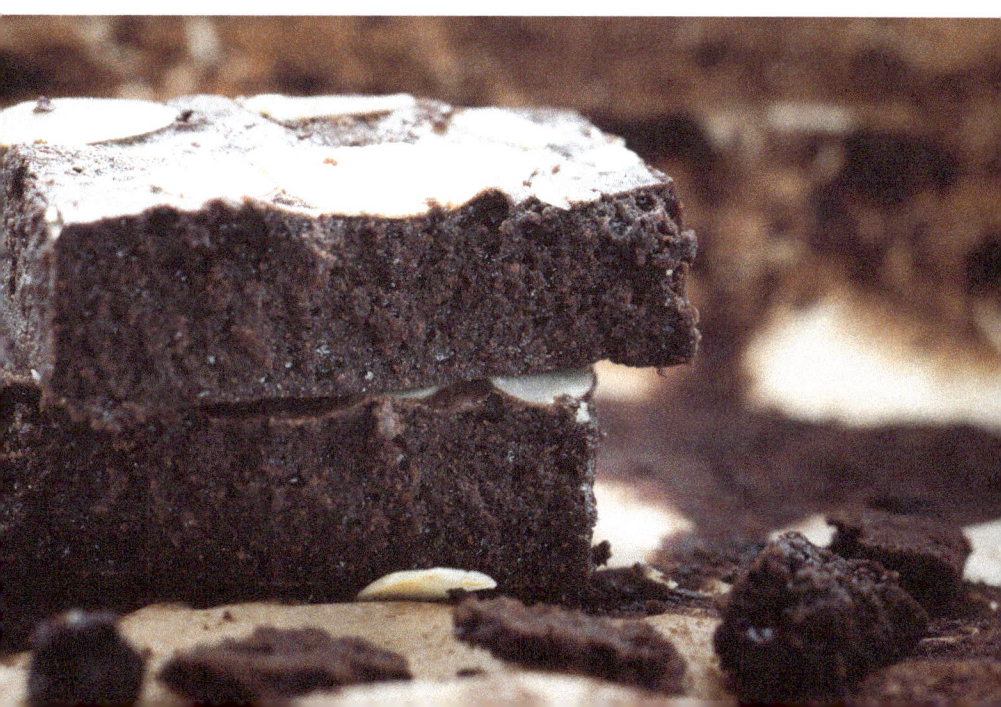

Anne Clark

Alfalfa Fudge

Makes 36

½ cup honey

½ cup peanut butter

½ tsp vanilla essence

pinch of grated citrus peel

¼ teaspoon cinnamon

¾ cup chopped alfalfa sprouts

1 cup soy milk powder

¼ cup carob powder

1. Put the honey in a saucepan and bring it to a boil. Boil for three minutes.
2. Pour the hot honey over the peanut butter and mix until smooth.
3. Add the vanilla, citrus peel, cinnamon and sprouts. Mix well.
4. Use your fingers to mix in a little of the soy milk powder and carob powder. Then knead in the remaining soy milk powder and carob powder.
5. Press the mixture into a greased lamington tin.
6. Chill and then cut into squares.

Variations: Instead of the soy milk powder, add ½ cup ground almond meal and ½ cup carob powder. You may also like to substitute another nut butter for part or all of the peanut butter. Flakes of coconut, wheatgerm, crushed nuts, seeds or grated carrots may be pressed on top of the mixture before it is chilled.

Alfalfa sprouts rich in alkaline minerals

Iron & calcium protect the body from infection

Great for the nerves

Celebration Cake

Serves 12

500 g pitted dates

500 g seedless raisins

125 g dried bananas

250 g almonds

1. Cut the dried bananas into small pieces.
2. Process all ingredients thoroughly in a food processor.
3. Press the mix firmly into a cake ring. Set aside to harden for an hour or so, then empty the cake onto a plate and slice.

Note: For a slightly softer texture, you may soak the dried fruits for a little while to expand the fruit. Drain the liquid and store for later use.

Dates – good for teeth

High calcium, magnesium, phosphorus, vitamin B1 & B5

Apple Crumble Pie

Serves 12

Base and topping:

½ cup walnuts, ground

4 tbsp dried sultanas

4 tsp tahini

4 tsp honey

½ tsp ground cinnamon

¼ cup ground almonds

½ cup sesame seeds

Filling:

6–7 apples sprinkled with lemon Juice

2 tbsp honey

½ cup raisins, chopped finely

1 tsp ground cinnamon

1 tsp vanilla essence

1. Mix together the base ingredients.
2. Set aside eight tablespoons for the topping.
3. Press the remaining mixture into a 23cm pie tin and chill.
4. Mix together the filling ingredients and pour into the pastry shell. Top with the reserved nut mixture.
5. Serve immediately with one of my ice cream delights.

Note: The base can be used as a sweet treat. Press into a tray, chill and wrap. Dried apples can be used in place of fresh which will extend the shelf life of crumble.

Walnuts – biotin = fat converting nutrient

Currants – high vitamin C

Apples – biotin, folic acid, vitamins A, C & E

Promotes good appetite

Overnight Fruit Tart

250 g dried figs

250 g dates

100 g sultanas

100 g brazil nuts

100 g walnuts

juice of 1 orange

shredded coconut

1. Mince dried fruit and nuts or place in food processor and process.
2. Add orange juice.
3. Sprinkle bottom of a 23cm pie dish with shredded coconut.
4. Press mass of fruit and nuts into pan.
5. Place in refrigerator overnight or for 4-5 hours.
6. Remove from pie dish and place on serving plate.
7. Slice into thin wedges to serve. Nice with nut cream or natural ice creams.

Figs – high iron & calcium

Source of manganese, copper, sodium, potassium, vitamin B1, B2 & B6

Prevents lung and chest ailments

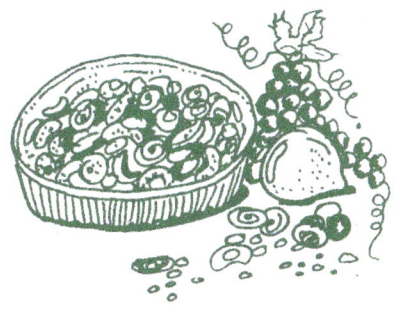

Delicious Mango Pie

Base:

½ cup hazelnuts, ground

½ cup almonds, ground

¼ cup coconut honey, enough to bind.

Filling:

6-7 ripe mangoes sliced into large pieces

2-3 tbsp orange juice

2–3 passionfruit

chopped nuts to top

1. Place base ingredients in a food processor and process until combined, adding enough honey to hold mass together.
2. Press into a prepared 23cm pie dish and set aside while preparing the filling:
3. Place mango in bowl with juice and passionfruit. Stir gently to combine.
4. Pour filling into base and refrigerate for 3–5 hours.
5. Serve with chopped nuts or grated coconut.

Mangoes – high carbohydrate

Vitamin A & potassium

High calories

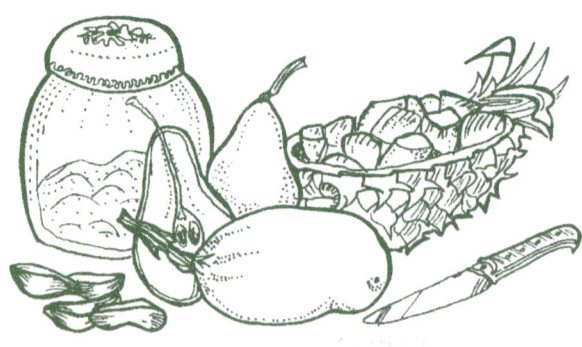

Raisin Truffles

Makes 12 small truffles

- 1 tbsp carob powder
- 1 tbsp tahini
- 1 tbsp water
- 50 g raisins
- 50 g oatmeal
- 25 g freshly grated coconut
- 1 tsp honey
- 1 tsp vanilla essence

1. Mix the carob powder, tahini and water together to form a smooth paste.
2. In a food processor, grind the raisins, oatmeal and coconut together.
3. Add the carob paste, honey and vanilla and mix again.
4. Divide the mixture into 12 small balls.
5. Roll in the grated coconut and refrigerate until required.

Carob – rich in B vitamins, calcium & phosphorus

Raisins – high potassium

Heart and muscle

Anne Clark

Pudding or Cake!

- 50 g mixed nuts
- 1 banana
- 125 g oats
- 1 tbsp wheatgerm
- 50 g raisins
- 2 tbsp apple juice concentrate
- 1 tsp ground cinnamon
- 1 tsp vanilla essence
- 1 tbsp poppy seeds
- 175 g fresh fruit (apples, pears, strawberries)

1. In a food processor or nut grinder, grind the nuts quite finely.
2. Reserve 2 strawberries for the garnish, then puree the banana and fresh fruit in a blender or food processor.
3. Mix the nuts and fruit with the remaining ingredients, until the mixture is moist but not sloppy. Add more oats if necessary.
4. Spoon the mixture into 500gm loaf tin, lined with greaseproof paper, and freeze for about two hours.
5. Turn out and serve in small pieces garnished with strawberries.

Bananas are high in potassium = stronger muscular system & healthy skin.

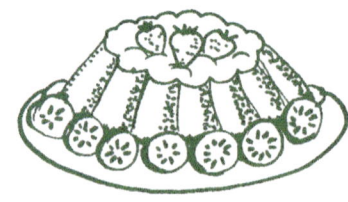

Crackle Pop!

Makes 24 slices

Although the honey and tahini are heated and the carob is melted for the topping, this slice is a real icebreaker for kids. It will make raw foods more exciting for them if you take it gradually. When you remove some of those high calorie cakes, sweets and ice creams, you need to have something to replace them with and Crackle Pop! does that for you. This slice is still high in calories but rich in carbohydrates, essential for energy and active people.

---

3 cups raw muesli

3 cups puffed rice cereal (not rice bubbles)

1–2 cups rolled oats

½ cup sesame seeds

½ cup sunflower seeds

½ cup pumpkin seed

½ cup dried peaches, chopped finely

250 g cocoa butter

¼ cup coconut paste

½ cup tahini

½ cup honey

1 cup carob buds

---

1. Melt the cocoa butter.

2. Combine all dry ingredients (muesli, puffed rice, oats, seeds and dried peaches) with melted cocoa butter in a large bowl. Mix together well.

3. Melt coconut paste with honey and tahini and combine thoroughly. Add to the wetted muesli mix.

4. Press mixture evenly over two lamington trays. Chill.

5. Top with melted carob.

6. Chill. Slice and wrap into individual serves.

This is a great energy bar for kids and adults

Pumpkin, sesame & sunflower seeds together = essential fatty acids

Banana Carob Cream

Makes 4–6 servings

5 pitted dates

½ cup raw cashews

2 tbsp carob powder

¾ cup water

1 tsp vanilla essence

5 ripe bananas

1. Put the dates, cashews, carob powder, water and vanilla into the container of a blender and puree.

2. Peel the bananas and cut them into chunks. With the blender running, add the banana chunks slowly until a thick puree is formed.

3. Pour the mixture into an ice cube tray and freeze until hard. Or serve immediately as a soft ice cream.

Dates & bananas are an important food for athletes

High in potassium

Ice Cream

2 cups soy milk powder

⅓ cup nuts

2 cups fruit or 1 cup carob powder

1 tsp lecithin granules

½ tsp kelp powder

1 tsp vanilla essence (optional)

1. Mix all together in your food processor or blender.

2. Freeze. Serve with fruit and nuts.

Lecithin rich in choline and inositol = utilisation of fats and cholesterol in the body.

In the Raw

Special Ice Cream

- 2 tbsp carob powder
- 1 tbsp date puree or prune puree
- 1 tbsp honey (optional)
- 1 tbsp almond or any nut butter
- 1 tsp vanilla essence
- 1 tbsp lemon juice
- 1 tsp cinnamon or 1 drop of essential oil of cinnamon
- 4–5 bananas (peeled and frozen)

1. Place all ingredients into a blender or food processor. Process until creamy.
2. Serve as a nutritious dessert or cream with fresh fruit. I like to have it simply as it is.

Note: To make date puree or prune puree, soak a quantity of dates in a little water (enough to cover) for several hours or overnight. Blend the fruit with soaking liquid and store in sterilised jars, in the refrigerator, with a little lemon juice until needed. The puree will generally keep for 3–4 weeks.

Rich in most vitamins & minerals

High calorie and high fibre

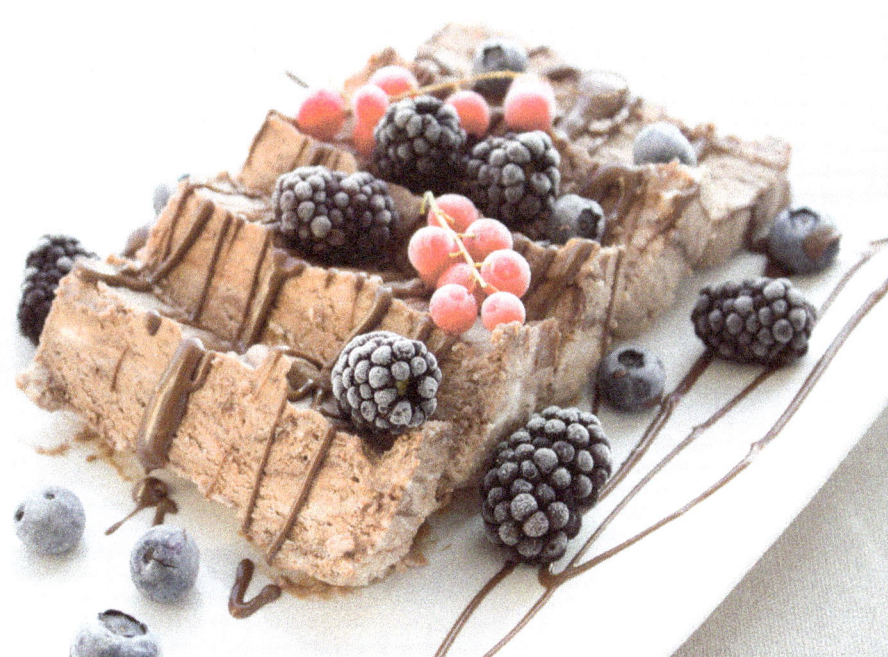

Raw Cashew Lemon/Lime Pie

Base:

250 g soaked raw almonds

½ cup dates

80 g raisins or sultanas

1 cup desiccated coconut

1 drop dōTERRA Cinnamon Bark essential oil

½ tsp vanilla essence

1 tsp agave syrup or pure honey

Filling:

320 g soaked cashews (soak in purified water for 24 hours, drain & put aside)

1 x 400 g tin coconut cream

½ tsp vanilla essence

5 drops dōTERRA Lemon or Lime essential oil

3 tbsp coconut oil

2 tbsp pure honey or agave syrup

Pinch of Himalayan salt or alternative

Sprinkle of nutmeg or cinnamon

Shredded coconut

1. Place all ingredients into a food processor and process until a mouldable consistency.
2. Press into a lightly oiled (coconut oil) pie base. For a thick base use the lot or, alternatively, roll any residue into balls.
3. Chill in freezer while preparing filling.
4. Place all ingredients into a food processor and process until the mix is creamy.
5. Add a little more essential oil to suit taste needs (remember, less is more in this case).
6. Pour the filling into the prepared pie shell and set in freezer for one hour.
7. Serve with sprinkle of nutmeg or cinnamon and shredded coconut.

High in essential fatty acids

High calorie and high protein

In the Raw

Cacao, Chia Seed & Coconut Cream Mousse

- 220 g cashews (soaked overnight)
- ½ cup dates (soaked overnight)
- 120 g cacao powder
- 60 g coconut oil
- 400 g tin of coconut cream
- 30–60 g honey
- 1 tsp coconut syrup
- 2 tbsp soaked chia seeds (5 mins soaking is fine)
- 10 drops Wild Orange essential oil
- Pinch of sea salt
- A few drops of vanilla essence

1. Blend all the main ingredients in a food processor until creamy and smooth.
2. Pour into mousse glass dishes and serve with sliced strawberries and coconut cream.

High in fibre and vitamin C

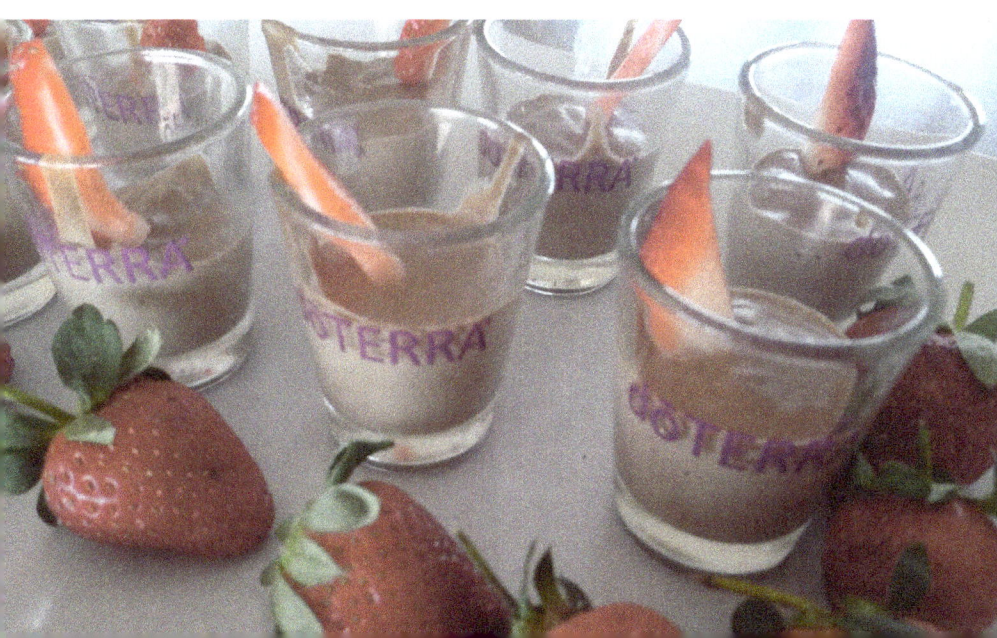

Anne Clark

Coconut Cream

1 cup coconut cream

½ cup dates (soaked overnight)

1 drop dōTERRA Cinnamon essential oil

1. Blend the coconut cream with dates and cinnamon oil
2. Serve with your desserts. Keeps in the fridge for a few days

High in essential fatty acids

Cacao Fruit & Nut Balls

1 cup unsweetened carob or cacao buds

2 cups soaked and drained almonds

1 cup desiccated coconut

1 cup sun-dried dates

1 cup sun-dried raisins or sultanas

1–2 tbsp honey

1–2 tbsp purified water

1 drop dōTERRA peppermint essential oil (optional)

1. In a food processor, grind the carob buds and almonds.
2. Add the dried fruit, coconut and honey and process, adding a little water and a few drops of essential oil to help with the binding and flavour, to suit your taste.
3. Scoop the mix out of the food processor, roll in coconut and shape into balls or press into a lightly oiled tray to slice into small squares later.
4. Store in the refrigerator and use as a healthy snack.

High in calcium and essential fatty acids

Recipes For the Family

Carob Apple Cake

Makes 12 slices

1½ cups sunflower seeds

4 tbsp carob powder

1 cup oat bran

½ cup fresh grated coconut

¾ cup dates, chopped finely

1 granny smith apple, chopped

1. Grind the sunflower seeds very finely.
2. Add the carob powder, oat bran and coconut and process to combine. Add the dates and chopped apple as the processor is in motion and be sure the mixture blends evenly.
3. Press mixture into a lightly greased tray or mould.
4. Serve with fresh tofu cream.

Calcium & magnesium and essential fatty acids

Tofu Cream

Makes 2 cups

300 g silken tofu

1 tbsp rice malt syrup

¼ cup dates, chopped

1 cup boiling water

1. Soak the dates for 30 minutes. Drain off some of the liquid (reserve for later use).
2. Process the tofu with syrup and date pulp.
3. Serve as a cream over the Carob Apple Cake.

Protein rich

Anne Clark

Apricot Fruit Spread

Makes 1½ cups

125 g dried apricots

60 g raisins

90 g dried apples

3½ cups orange juice

1. Combine all ingredients in a large saucepan and simmer over a gentle heat until fruit is soft.
2. Puree the mixture in a blender and pour into sterilised jars.
3. When cool, seal and store in the refrigerator.

Vitamin A and calcium

High fibre

Use as an alternative to jam

Date Pecan Rolls

Makes 12–15 rolls

2 cups dates, chopped

½ cup pecan nuts, chopped

½ cup coconut

1. Place dates and nuts into a food processor and process until combined.
2. Form into rolls or balls and roll in coconut.

Protein enriched

essential fatty acids

In the Raw

Peach Nibbles

Makes 12–15 balls or 12 slices

¾ cup dried peaches, chopped

¾ cup coconut, shredded

1 tsp lemon peel, grated

1 tsp orange peel, grated

1 tbsp orange juice extra shredded coconut

1. Cover dried peaches with boiling water and stand for 20 minutes. Drain off liquid.
2. Mince peaches and mix in lightly with coconut in food blender.
3. Add remaining ingredients.
4. Knead until well mixed. If mixture is too dry add more orange juice. If mixture is too wet, add more coconut.
5. Shape into small balls and roll in coconut. Refrigerate.

High vitamin C & vitamin A

Great energy slice

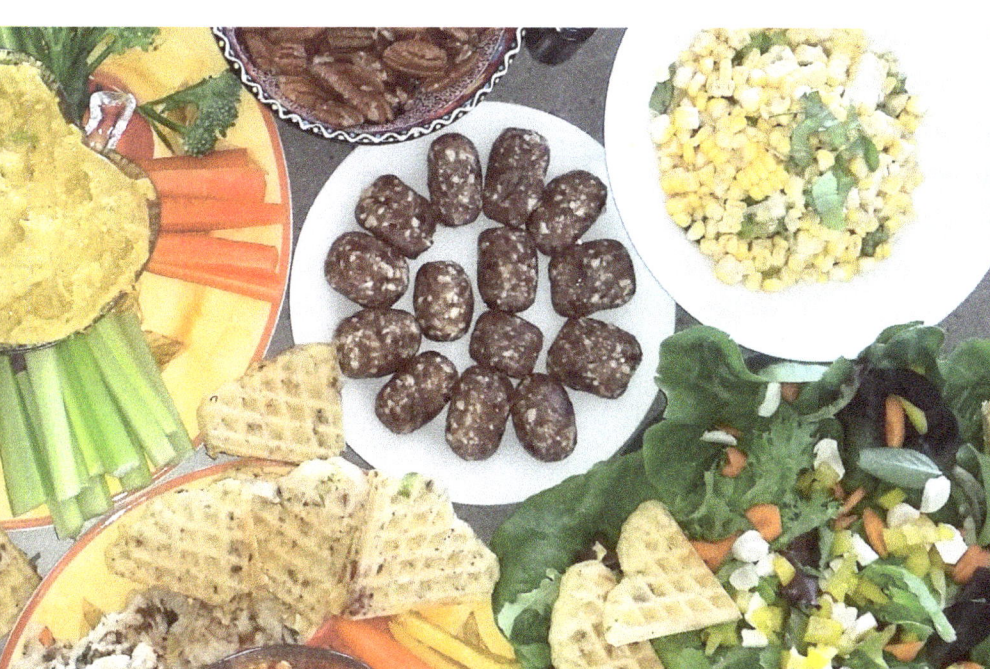

Anne Clark

Prune Bars

Makes 18 small balls or 12 slices

⅔ cup prunes, finely chopped

⅓ cup dried apple, finely chopped

1 tbsp sunflower seeds

1 tbsp sesame seeds

1 cup rolled oats

1 cup almonds, in their skins

½ cup soy milk powder

1 tbsp rice bran syrup or honey

⅓ cup orange juice

2 tsp lemon peel, grated

1. Combine all dry ingredients into a food processor and process to combine.
2. Add dried apple, juice, syrup and lemon peel and process until mixture sticks together. Add extra juice if necessary.
3. Press into a foil lined 20cm x 30cm slice tin. Refrigerate.
4. Cut into squares and serve as a treat.

Note: Replace prunes with dates, pears or figs for a sweeter more concentrated taste.

Protein enriched and high fibre

Low fat

Essential fatty acids

In the Raw

Bumpy Carob Slice

Makes 12–15 balls or 12 slices

2 cups rolled oats

3 tsp prune juice

1 cup almonds, in their skins

2 tbsp carob powder

1 cup dates, chopped finely

extra juice to bind

1 cup sultanas sprinkle of coconut

1. Combine all ingredients into a food processor. Process until the mixture begins to stick together.
2. Press into a foil lined 20cm x 30cm slice tin. Refrigerate.
3. Cut into squares when the slice has set.

Good for skin and bowel stimulation

Rich in minerals

Lazy Salad

Shredded lettuce

3 mushrooms, sliced

1 red capsicum

1 green capsicum

1 cucumber, sliced

hand full of mung bean sprouts

dash of Bragg Liquid Aminos

1. Seed and slice the capsicums.
2. Add to remaining ingredients and drizzle a little Bragg Liquid Aminos over the top.
3. Serve with Almond Sunflower Spread.

High in chlorophyll, vitamin C and protein

Anne Clark

Gazpacho Soup

Serves 3

- 2 tomatoes, quartered and cored
- 1–2 tbsp fresh parsley, chopped
- 1 cucumber, peeled and sliced
- 1 small onion, quartered
- 1 green capsicum, sliced
- 3 cups tomato juice
- ⅓ cup apple cider or red wine vinegar or alternative *
- 1 tbsp olive oil (optional)
- dash of Bragg Liquid Aminos *

1. Place all ingredients into a blender and blend for one minute or until combined.
2. Serve cold over chopped cucumbers and tomatoes. Delicious!

*Note: An alternative to cider vinegar or red wine vinegar is mirin rice wine or very diluted lemon juice.

Bragg Liquid Aminos is a seasoning formula by Paul C. Bragg, one of America's health pioneers and originator of health food stores. It is made from soybeans and purified water and is a gourmet replacement for tamari and soy sauce. It has no preservatives, is not fermented and contains no colouring agents, additives, alcohol or chemicals. The best news is that Bragg Liquid Aminos is not heated and is Kosher certified. It is available from most health food shops.

Rich in minerals

Natural aid to digestion

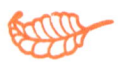

In the Raw

Almond Sunflower Spread

- 1 cup whole almonds
- 1 cup sunflower seeds
- 1 small carrot, finely grated
- juice of 1 lemon
- ¼ cup purified water
- ¼ cup eggless mayonnaise
- ½ cup parsley finely chopped
- 2 tbsp tamari sauce
- 4 cloves garlic, minced
- ⅛ tsp cayenne pepper
- 1 tsp cumin or coriander
- 1 tsp marjoram

1. Place almonds and sunflower seeds in a medium-sized bowl and cover with water. Allow to soak for six hours. Drain, rinse and drain again.
2. In a food processor, blend almonds and sunflower seeds for 30 seconds. Add remaining ingredients and process until smooth.
3. Cover and chill before serving.

Great for circulation, inflammation and painful joints

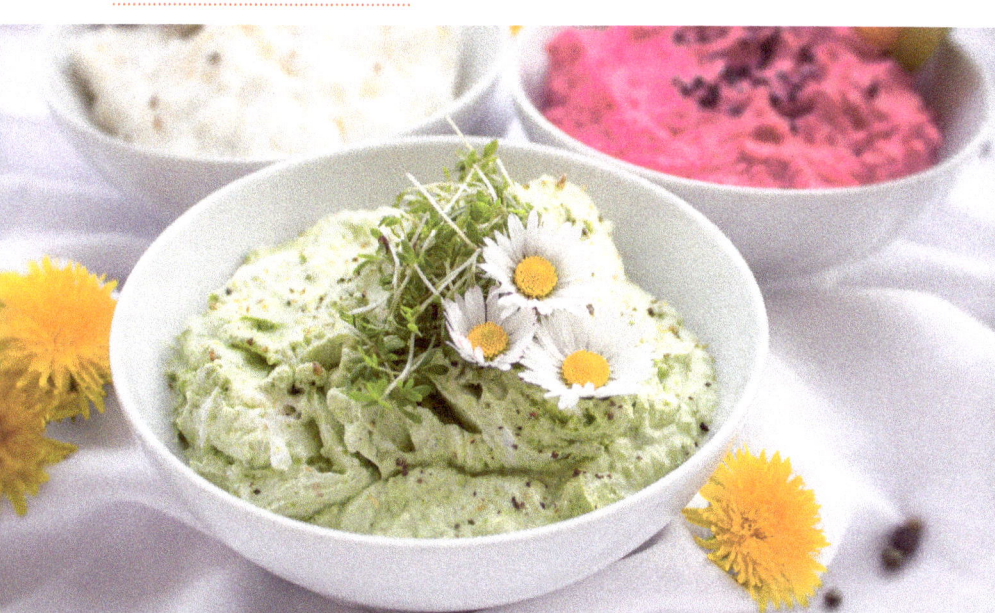

Anne Clark

Savoury Rice Waffles

Makes about 15 waffles

3 cups cooked brown rice

½ cup cornflour (maize)

2 cups brown rice flour

1 tbsp egg replacer or alternative

vegetable seasoning broth powder *

2½ cups of water or veg stock

1 tbsp olive oil

seasonings of your choice

1. Combine all the dry ingredients and mix well.
2. Add liquids and stir in to combine. Add more liquid if mixture is too thick. Mixture should be of pancake consistency.
3. Drop three tablespoons of mixture per waffle mould and spread out evenly.
4. Cook for 8–10 minutes per waffle.
5. Serve with Almond Sunflower Spread and salad.

Free from gluten and eggs

Wholemeal Waffles

- 3 cups of plain wholemeal flour
- ½ cup soy flour
- ½ cup polenta (corn meal)
- ¼ cup linseed
- 1 tsp vegetable seasoning broth powder *
- ½ cup sesame seeds
- 4–5 cups warm water
- 1 tbsp olive oil
- dash of pepper

1. Mix all dry ingredients together.
2. Add liquids and stir in extra seasoning if necessary Add more water if mixture is too thick.
3. Lightly grease a hot waffle iron.
4. Spoon in the desired amount of mixture and cook for approx. 7–8 minutes.
5. Serve with your favourite dip and salad.

*Note: Vegetable seasoning broth powder (Nature's Sunshine) is used as a seasoning or as a tasty broth. With a blend of 23 vegetables, herbs and spices in a convenient 255gm container, each serve is fat free and nutritious with only 42 kJ. Available at most health food stores.

Rich in B-complex vitamins and essential fatty acids.

Anne Clark

Oat Waffles

- 3–4 cups rolled oats
- ½ cup polenta (corn meal)
- 1 cup wholemeal flour
- ½ cup soy flour
- 1 tbsp olive oil
- 1 tsp mixed dried herbs
- handful of fresh, chopped herbs
- ¼ cup poppy seeds
- 4–5 cups water
- 1 clove garlic, crushed

1. Mix all dry ingredients well.
2. Combine with wet ingredients, adding more water if necessary. You can process the oats before combining with other ingredients for a finer waffle.
3. Cook in a hot waffle iron for eight minutes.
4. Serve with salad.

Wheat, egg & dairy free

Great for fussy eaters

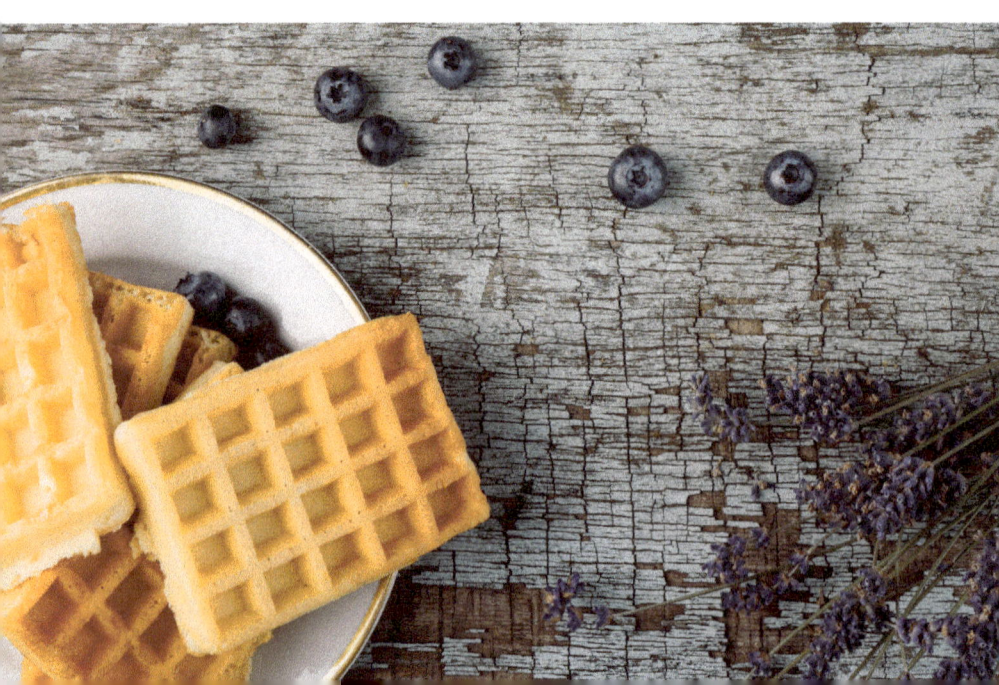

In the Raw

Spark Up Drink

Makes 2 large serves

4 large carrots

½ small beetroot

1 clove garlic

1 stalk of celery

1 tsp grated ginger

4 leaves of sorrel (optional)

3 spinach leaves

1 stalk of parsley

20 blades of wheatgrass (optional)

½ tsp slippery elm powder

1. Juice all ingredients in a juicer and drink immediately for freshness and flavour, and to provide you with vitamins, minerals and enzymes for the whole day.

Calcium & magnesium

Great for students

Grain Drink

Makes 2 large serves

1 cup coarsely ground oats, wheat or other grains

2 cups water

1 tbsp almond or nut butter

2 tbsp honey juice of 1 lemon

2 bananas

⅓ tsp cinnamon and ground cloves

1. Soak ground grains overnight in water.

2. Next morning, strain grains and blend liquid together with other ingredients.

3. Add vanilla and ginger to taste.

Silica – the skin mineral

A drink for memory and alertness

Anne Clark

Apple and Beetroot Juice

Makes 2 serves

This sparkling red juice has many cancer-reducing benefits. Apples have the malic and tartaric acids and inhibit growth of ferments and disease-producing bacteria. Pectin removes the residues of radiation. Beet juice is one of the most valuable juices for helping to build up the red corpuscles in the blood, while also helping to cleanse the liver. Lemon juice will stimulate the liver to produce enzymes. The lemon's antimicrobial and mucus-resolving action make it beneficial in the formation of bile, the absorption of minerals, cleansing of the blood and elimination of parasite infestation.

2 apples, peeled and cored	1. Cut the apples and beet into pieces and juice together with the lemon and rind.
½ medium beetroot	2. Serve in fancy glasses and garnish with a slice of strawberry.
½ medium lemon	
1 strawberry	*Blood cleansing liver drink*

Almond Sultana Slice

- 1 cup almonds, in their skins
- 1 cup puffed rice cereal
- 1 cup coconut
- 2 cups quick cook oats
- 2 tbsp soy milk powder
- ¼ tsp cinnamon
- 1 cup sultanas
- ½ cup sunflower seeds
- 5 tbsp honey
- ½ cup boiling water

1. Place almonds and puffed rice cereal into a food processor and process until mixture resembles a meal consistency.
2. Add remaining ingredients except for water and process until combined.
3. Add water as a very last binding ingredient and process until you have a mixture which can be pressed into a suitable tray or rolled into balls.
4. Refrigerate for an hour or more.

Calcium & silica

Relieves fatigue – high in energy

Anne Clark

Pawpaw Sultana Slice

3–4 cups rolled oats

1 cup coconut

½ cup dried pawpaw, chopped finely

1 cup sultanas

3–4 tbsp honey

1 tbsp soy milk powder

1 cup water

¼ tsp cinnamon

1. Process the rolled oats in a food processor.
2. Add coconut, dried fruits and process until the mixture has combined.
3. Add soy milk powder, cinnamon and honey while the processor is in motion. Add enough water to bind.
4. Press the mixture into a lightly greased tray or mould and allow to set in the refrigerator.

High fibre and cleansing abilities

Flax Seed Pudding

⅓ cup flax seed, freshly ground

2 tbsp ground almond meal

1 tbsp soy milk powder

1 banana

1 apple, grated

juice of 1 orange

1 tbsp honey or maple syrup

2 cups water

1. Add boiling water to ground flax seed, almond meal and soy milk powder. Place in a heavy-duty food processor or Vitamix and process. Add banana, apple, orange juice and honey and process further until mixture thickens.

2. Alternatively, bring water to boil, add ground flax seed, stirring constantly to avoid lumps. Let boil for approximately two minutes or until mixture starts to thicken. Let cool completely. Stir in nuts, fruit and honey.

3. Chill and serve.

The Rolls Royce of puddings

High in fibre and great nutrition for all especially babies & fussy toddlers.

Anne Clark

Raw Cashew Cream Slice

Base:

2 cups macadamia nuts, blended

1 cup cashews blended

½ cup chopped dates

1 tbsp orange juice extra water to bind.

1. Process the macadamia nuts with the cashews until the mixture resembles a breadcrumb consistency.
2. Add the chopped dates while processor is still motoring along.
3. Add orange juice and just enough water to bind the mixture.
4. Press this mixture into an oiled glass rectangular or pie dish to form your wholesome base. Set aside in the freezer while you prepare your filling.

Filling:

3 cups raw cashews (soaked in oxygenated purified water)

½ cup pure honey

½ cup coconut oil

½ cup lemon juice or juice of one lemon (reserve some)

1–2 tsp vanilla essence

1. Soak the cashews in purified water overnight or for several hours until nuts are expanded and full of water. Drain off the excess water and process in the food processor.
2. Melt honey and coconut oil and add to cashew mixture. Continue to process as you add the remaining ingredients. When you get to the lemon juice, reserve a little in case you have too much liquid.
3. Process the cashew mixture thoroughly until nice and creamy and smooth.
4. Pour into the prepared pie base and chill in fridge.

In the Raw

Topping:

1 cup dates

1 cup frozen mixed berries

1 cup boiling water

1. Soak the dates in one cup of boiling water. When it cools, drain off a little of the liquid.

2. Blend the dates with frozen berries until it forms a puree.

3. Serve a dollop over each slice of cashew cream slice. Delicious! This topping will keep for a week in the refrigerator and in the freezer for three months. We never have it around that long though because everyone loves it.

Brain food!

Essential fatty acids and high protein

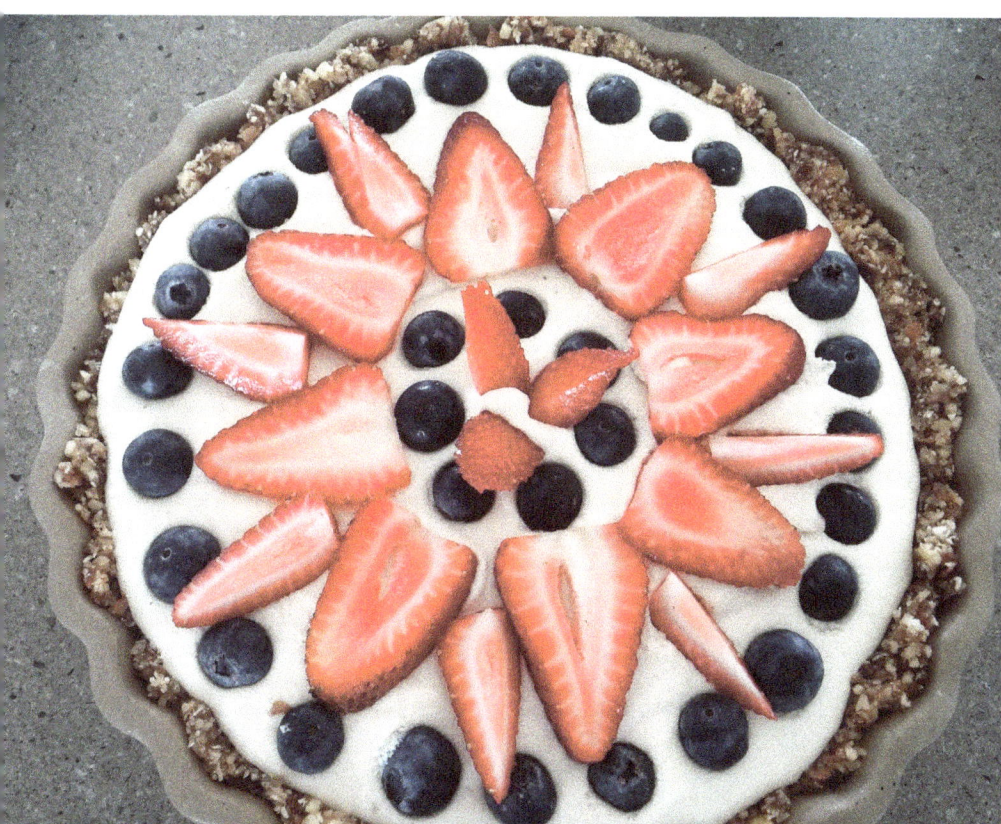

Anne Clark

Carob Date Balls

- 1¼ cups unsweetened carob buds
- 1 tsp coconut syrup
- 3 cups rolled oats
- 1 tsp vanilla essence
- 1 cup chopped dates
- 1 cup sultanas or raisins
- 2 tbsp honey
- 1 cup coconut
- water to bind ingredients (lemongrass or chamomile tea is also excellent to add as your liquid to bind)

1. Process the carob buds and oats together.
2. Gradually add the dates, sultanas, coconut, honey and liquid until you have a mixture that you can roll into balls or press into an oiled lamington tray.
3. Roll the balls in a little coconut or crushed nuts and serve chilled with fresh strawberries. Delicious when sliced up into squares and eaten as a snack between meals. Enjoy.

High protein treat

High calcium

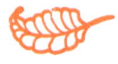

In the Raw

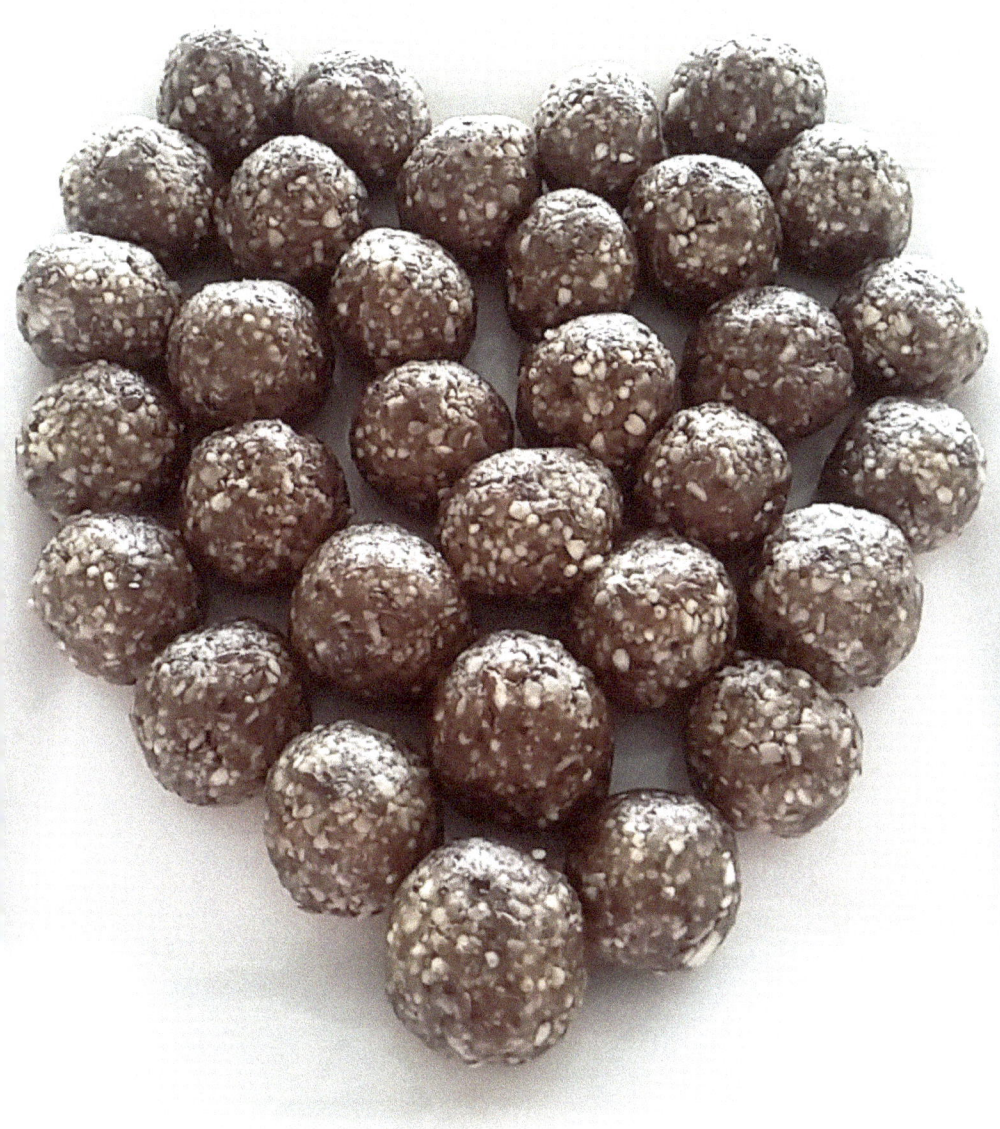

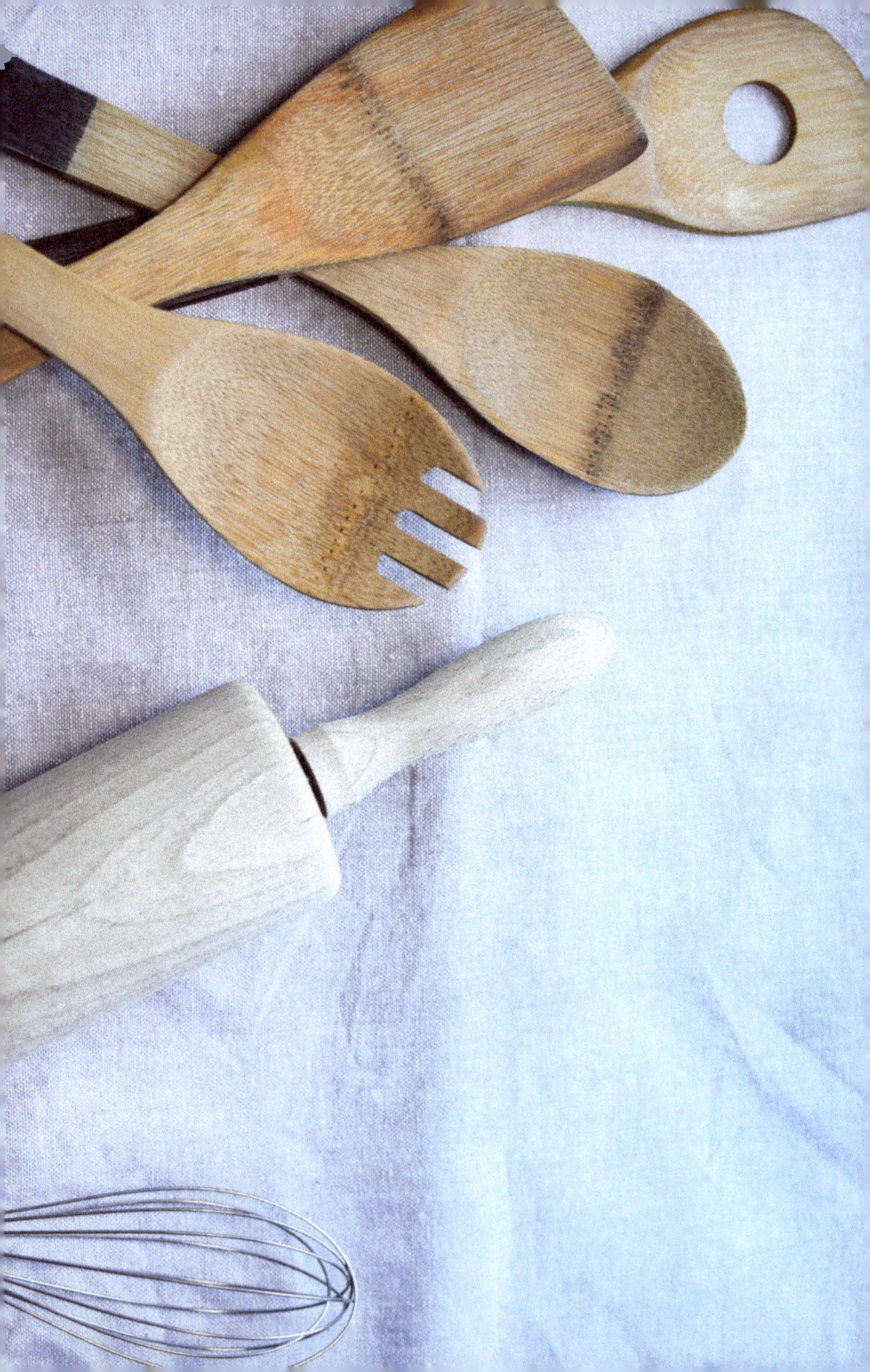

 # Cooking tips

- For greasing baking trays and glass dishes I use a combination of coconut oil, olive oil and macadamia oil, or any one of these oils on their own.

- Always add less of required liquid suggested in recipes at first, because you can always add more if needed instead of spoiling your recipe with too much liquid.

- Blend leftover salad greens and vegies with a little tahini, nut paste, avocado or seeds, and make a pate or dip. Season with soy sauce.

- Rinse your food processor after using with fresh water and keep the rinse water as vegetable stock. It is far better the vegetable scraps are used in future creations rather than blocking your sink.

- Limit the use of flavourings and condiments so you can appreciate the real flavours of your food.

- Think ahead when making dishes like Hazelnut Loaf and Avocado Supreme. Will the remaining leftover portions be used the next day? If not, do not bother keeping leftovers as these will not keep very long. These dishes are ideal for parties.

- Make use of your food processor by grinding nuts and grating vegetables ahead of time. Quite often this will cut down food preparation in the long run.

- Freeze orange wedges to serve as a healthy ice block for children. You can also freeze lemon, lime and orange juice in ice cube trays and use for preparing sweet sauces or for serving with fruit salads.

- Avoid buying fruit and vegetables sealed in plastic bags as they become bruised and deteriorate without air. Mushrooms are especially vulnerable and should not be bought if displayed in sealed plastic bags.

- Keep wholemeal flour and wheatgerm in the refrigerator during hot weather. Never put new flour on top of old.

- Lemon juice is easily applied to fruit slices if you put it in a spray bottle.

- Store dried fruit, flour, pulses, rice and spices in cool, dry conditions. They will keep longer in dark jars.

- Vanilla extract or essence recipe:
  1 vanilla bean
  ¼ cup water
  ¼ tsp lecithin (optional)
  2 tsp honey
  2 tsp vegetable oil

- Cut up vanilla bean into small pieces and place in bowl, then pour boiling water over. Cover the bowl and allow mixture to stand overnight. Grind mixture in blender, strain and return juice to blender. Add lecithin (optional) and honey and vegetable oil. Blend mixture and pour into a bottle. Store in refrigerator.

- Excess fruit need not be discarded as you can slice and freeze portions of the fruit and use in whips, smoothies and frozen fruit pies.

- Dried herbs are stronger than fresh. Use half the amount of dried to replace fresh herbs in a recipe.

- Onions should be stored in the refrigerator. Peel under cold running water and slice, dice or puree quickly in food processor. Store chopped onion in sealed container in the refrigerator for general use for up to one week. Keep juice for dressings, etc.

- Place an inverted saucer on the bottom of the salad bowl. This stops the dressing forming a pool and making the salad soggy. Always dress a salad just before serving. Don't use too much dressing.

- Do not store oranges & lemons together or both will become mouldy.

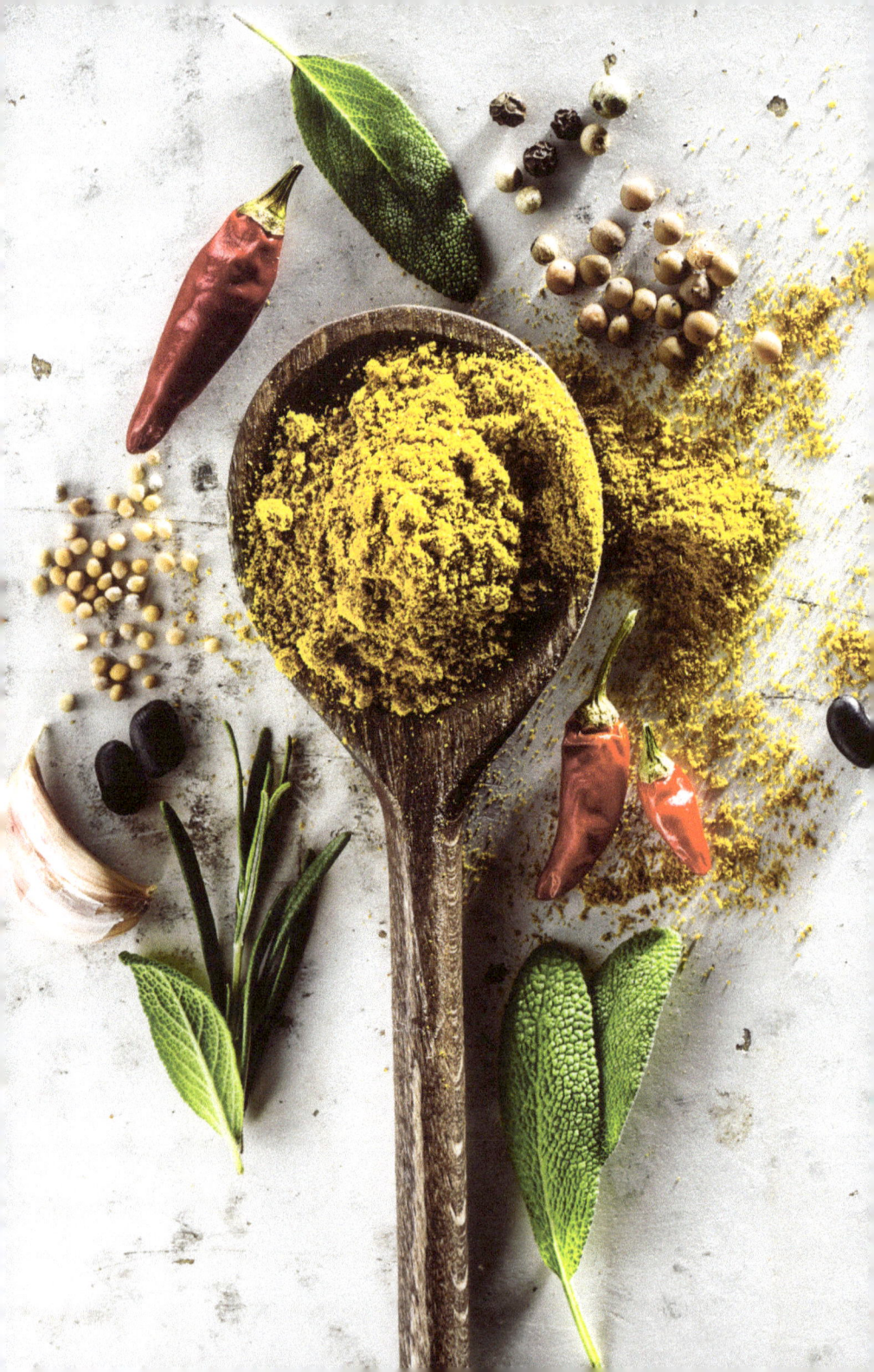

 # Ingredients in detail

When I look through other recipe books, I am often disappointed when I come across an ingredient that I know nothing about, so for your benefit I have listed all the ingredients used in this book with an appropriate explanation to go with it. I hope you find this helpful and informative.

FRUITS & VEGETABLES

There are so many fruits and vegetables available to us today. Sometimes that can be a good thing, but I feel it also leads to a slight off balance when it comes to our health. We are quite often eating fruits and vegetables which are not native to our area and out of season. This can harm our body harmony; maybe not quite as much as consuming sugar or cooked foods, but over a period of time it will make a difference. Try to consume fruits and vegetables in their correct season and when they are at their peak. Once fruit and vegetables are cut, their keeping time decreases and the food should be covered to keep the cut surface moist and prevent aromas in the refrigerator.

Most fruits and vegetables are high in B-complex vitamins, vitamins C and E, and minerals. Refer to the Vitamins and Minerals section for more details on the nutritional qualities of fruit and vegetables.

Dietary fibre comes in many different forms. The kinds of fibre in fruits and vegetables not only prevent constipation but also have the potential to help control blood sugar and cholesterol levels.

Following are most of the fruits and vegetables I use in this book, and of course there are many more.

Fruits: Apple, banana, mango, passionfruit, peach, grape, raspberry, strawberry, blueberry, pawpaw, pineapple, mandarin, starfruit, orange, lemon, lime, grapefruit, plum, nectarine, kiwi fruit, melon, avocado.

Vegetables: Brussels sprout, carrot, celery, cucumber, spinach, shallots, mushroom, beetroot, tomato, corn, snow pea, pumpkin, zucchini, cherry tomato, turnip, potato, sweet potato, watercress, broccoli, cauliflower, capsicum, cabbage, radish, asparagus, lettuce.

SPROUTS

Sprouts are a complete food. They can be grown by anyone, anytime and anywhere. I sprout mung beans at home, because they are the easiest and most convenient for me personally. All you need is a plastic container, water and the seeds. I place a quantity of beans in the base of my flat container. Cover with water. Rinse after 24 hours. Allow the beans to stand for 12 hours, rinse again and repeat for 2–3 days. When you are happy with the sprout length and form, store in the refrigerator. See Sprouts section for more information.

Sprouts: alfalfa, aduki beans, lentil, soy bean, mung bean, wheat.

NUTS AND SEEDS

When buying nuts make sure they are really fresh. The rancid oils in old nuts are harmful to the stomach, retard the secretion of pancreatic enzymes and destroy vitamins. Nuts are best stored in your refrigerator for up to several months. Shelled nuts should be bought in much smaller quantities and they too should be refrigerated. Vary your nuts so that you get a good balance of essential amino acids. Nuts are high in protein and natural digestible fats. Never combine nuts with meat.

Nut protein is better value than the usual alternative of a piece of meat, poultry or fish, depending of course on your accessibility to such produce. When obtained raw, nuts supply generous amounts of easily assimilated protein, minerals and vitamins, and an excellent supply of essential unsaturated fatty acids.

A mixture of almonds, Brazil and cashew nuts will supply all the required daily protein and still not exceed the recommended daily fat intake.

These are some of the nuts that I have used in my recipes.

Nuts: Brazil nut, pecan, walnut, almond, cashew, pine nut, peanut, hazelnut, coconut (nut of the tropics).

Also, don't miss out on the wonderful advantages of **seeds** in your diet. The three seeds which provide an ideal combination of protein and essential fatty acids are: sunflower, pumpkin and sesame. The other seeds which I use are poppyseed, linseed and celery seed.

HERBS AND SPICES

I can't imagine what it would be like if we never acquainted ourselves with the usefulness of herbs and spices. I have only used a limited number of herbs and spices, but I urge you to explore the potential of all the remaining types available. Always buy spices and dried herbs in small quantities. Try grinding your own spices for the wonderful aromas and tastes.

The nutrient content of herbs can be used on a day-to-day basis. Take parsley for example; not only is it an excellent source of magnesium and the mineral calcium, but daily use of parsley can help your nerves. Parsley is one of the richest sources of potassium – the muscle mineral – as well as iron and vitamin C, which work in combination to incinerate waste matter within the body. Iron transports oxygen to every cell of the body and vitamin C helps the function along.

These are the herbs and spices that I have used in this book.

Herbs: Parsley, mint, basil, dill, fennel, chives, celery powder, garlic, coriander, caraway, curry powder, tarragon, chilli, ginger, cumin, sage, mustard, thyme, oregano.

Spices: Nutmeg, cinnamon, cloves.

DRIED FRUITS

Dried fruits are a highly concentrated food and should be eaten sparingly. Dried fruits have a high ratio of simple sugars and that makes them an ideal energy food. Be sure to buy sun-dried fruit only. Avoid sulphur-dried fruit. Unsulphured fruit will be darker, chewier, and devoid of the negative effects of added sulphur. Avoid honey-dipped or sugared dried fruit. Soak dried fruits for easier digestion and keep the juice and use it in fruit sauces or smoothies.

Dried fruits include: Apples, apricots, bananas, currants, raisins, figs, mangoes, paw paws, peaches, pears, pineapple rounds, plums and grapes.

SWEETENERS AND FLAVOURINGS

On a natural diet, sweeteners become a product of the past, however natural sweeteners can be incorporated into your diet, in moderation.

Honey is a food that should be consumed with great respect and awe as it takes a bee its entire lifetime to make one teaspoon of honey. Honey is primarily a simple carbohydrate, which is absorbed rapidly into the bloodstream, immediately raising the blood sugar level.

Vanilla essence or extract is achieved by soaking the vanilla bean in water or alcohol. Imitation vanilla is a product of synthetic, chemical ingredients and is not recommended. See a natural recipe for vanilla in the Cooking Tips section.

Liquid malt is a thick, sweet syrup made by fermenting barley or other grains with yeast.

Carob is a powder that is ground from the pods of the evergreen carob tree. Carob, unlike chocolate, contains a negligible amount of fat, no caffeine and encourages, rather than inhibits, absorption of calcium. Carob contains calcium, phosphorus and iron.

Apple juice concentrate is rich in vitamin C and makes an excellent natural sweetener in place of sugar.

Vegetable stock is achieved by steaming vegetables and reserving the juice left behind. You can add onion juice and finely grated vegetables to the stock to enrich the flavour. It should be stored in the refrigerator.

Miso is a paste made from fermented soy beans. There are different varieties according to the different grains used to mix with the miso during fermentation. Only use a small amount at a time. Store in the refrigerator.

Tamari (soy sauce) is a wheat-free soy sauce derived from the liquid of miso production. It adds flavour and colour to vegetable and salad dressings and dips. It should also be used sparingly. However, it is far better than commercially produced soy sauce available in the supermarket, which is very high in salt and can raise blood pressure.

Soya mayonnaise is another product from the soya bean. You will need to check labels in health food shops, as some brands of soya mayonnaise have sugar and eggs added to them. You can make your own by blending a small amount of tofu with tamari and lemon juice.

Brewer's yeast and torula yeast vary a little in their nutrient properties. Torula is low in sodium and is best suited for people with hypertension or any other problem related to a high sodium (salt) intake. Torula also has approximately double the fibre and calcium content than brewer's yeast. Brewer's yeast is higher in magnesium. Some people may prefer the stronger taste of torula, while others will prefer the slightly sweeter and saltier taste of brewer's yeast. If you have allergies to fungal foods, avoid yeast, and look to concentrated foods for B vitamins.

NUT AND SEED BUTTERS

Almond butter, peanut butter, cashew butter, sunflower butter and sesame butter (tahini) are made by blending the raw nut or seed with either a little water or olive oil until a paste is formed. Store blended nut and seed butters in the refrigerator until required. Tahini can be stored in the pantry for short periods of time.

Get used to using these nutritious alternatives to butter. **Avocado** can also be used as a suitable spread and should be included in an all-raw diet. Although avocados are primarily a fruit they are able to combine with most vegetables. The flesh of one avocado blended with one tablespoon of lemon juice and a half teaspoon of kelp can transform a salad into a masterpiece or make a simple spread over crackers or bread. With sprouts this will be a completely balanced meal. Try it sometime if you haven't already.

FATS & OILS

If you must use oil, then **olive oil** is probably the best. I also use **coconut oil**, **macadamia oil**, **avocado oil**, **safflower oil** and **hemp oil**. These oils provide a richer flavour. It is not necessary to add oil to your diet, even though I have used it in some of my recipes. You would be better off to eat whole foods like avocado, nuts and seeds to get the essential fatty acids.

Shredded coconut is easily created by grating the coconut pulp. You can dry the coconut out in the sun and store in the refrigerator. Coconut is best eaten on its own or with other fruits.

FLOUR & GRAINS

Flour is basically ground grain, suitable for baking nourishing breads, cookies and cakes. The most popular varieties are **wheat, rye, corn and buckwheat**, as well as **soya beans**. Freshly ground is best. The resulting flour will be slightly coarser but will still be adequate for all forms of baking and will taste better in the finished product. I caution everyone about consuming foods with flour as the major ingredient, because as soon as you process the grain you change the structure of the food and too much grain in the diet can be very mucus forming.

Rolled oats are richly nutritious. They are high in protein, contain polyunsaturated fats, a little vitamin E, and plenty of the B-complex vitamins and most minerals. When you think of oats, think of them lowering high blood cholesterol and regulating blood fats. For oatmeal simply blend rolled oats in your food processor.

EXTRAS

Tofa (bean curd) is a high protein food made from soy beans that can be used in savoury and sweet dishes. The two main types are the Chinese (dow-foo) and the Japanese (tofu), with the latter usually being sweeter. Sold generally in custard form, tofu will keep for one week in refrigerator. Keep tofu immersed in cold water and change the water daily. Although a cooked food, a little tofu incorporated into a raw food diet will not hurt and will give your diet variety.

Soy milk is made from the soya bean and is an ideal alternative to cow's milk. Some soy milks contain malt that is derived from barley. These may not be tolerated by some coeliacs. Other soy milks contain rice malt and these are suitable for a gluten-free diet.

Muesli is best eaten at midday. Why? Well, traditionally muesli is consumed as a breakfast cereal, but remember that I said it is far better to start the day with fruit juice or fruit because it takes less energy to digest and process in the body than grain. Muesli is usually poorly combined and therefore taxing on the digestive system.

Agar agar is a Japanese seaweed setting agent. Use as a substitute for gelatine. It is sold in packets as powder and flakes and in blocks of fine strands.

Kelp is a brown seaweed powder with a high nutritional value. Use in dips and sprinkle over salad greens. The chemical composition of human blood is said to be very similar to seawater and by obtaining seafood, the balance of nutrients is most suitable for effective absorption. The strong taste of kelp is due to the abundance of nutrients. When properly prepared and served, a kelp meal will provide good protein value, nearly all minerals and vitamins and, for total vegetarians (actually anyone), the essential vitamin B12.

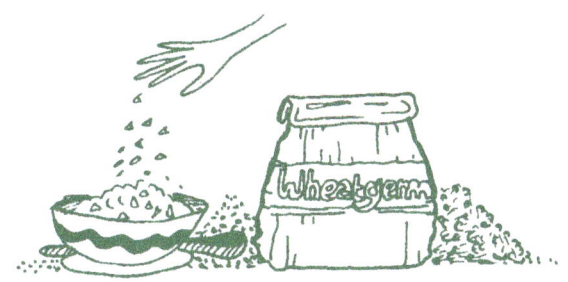

Wheatgerm is high in vitamin E and a good source of vitamin B6. Sprinkle over fruit or combine with smoothies. Never heat wheatgerm or associated products, as heating destroys these vitamins.

HOW & WHEN TO BUY

First of all, freshness is of utmost importance and, obviously, you should only buy food and ingredients when you need them. In storage, fruits and vegetables lose their nutrient content rapidly, so buy wisely and think about what you will be eating the day before if possible. Seek out markets that you know supply organic fruits and vegetables. Consider forming a group of likeminded people and buy nuts, seeds and grains in bulk as you will save a lot of money this way.

Remember, ingredients make up your food and food is your fuel. Make sure your fuel is the best you can get and you will reap the benefits!

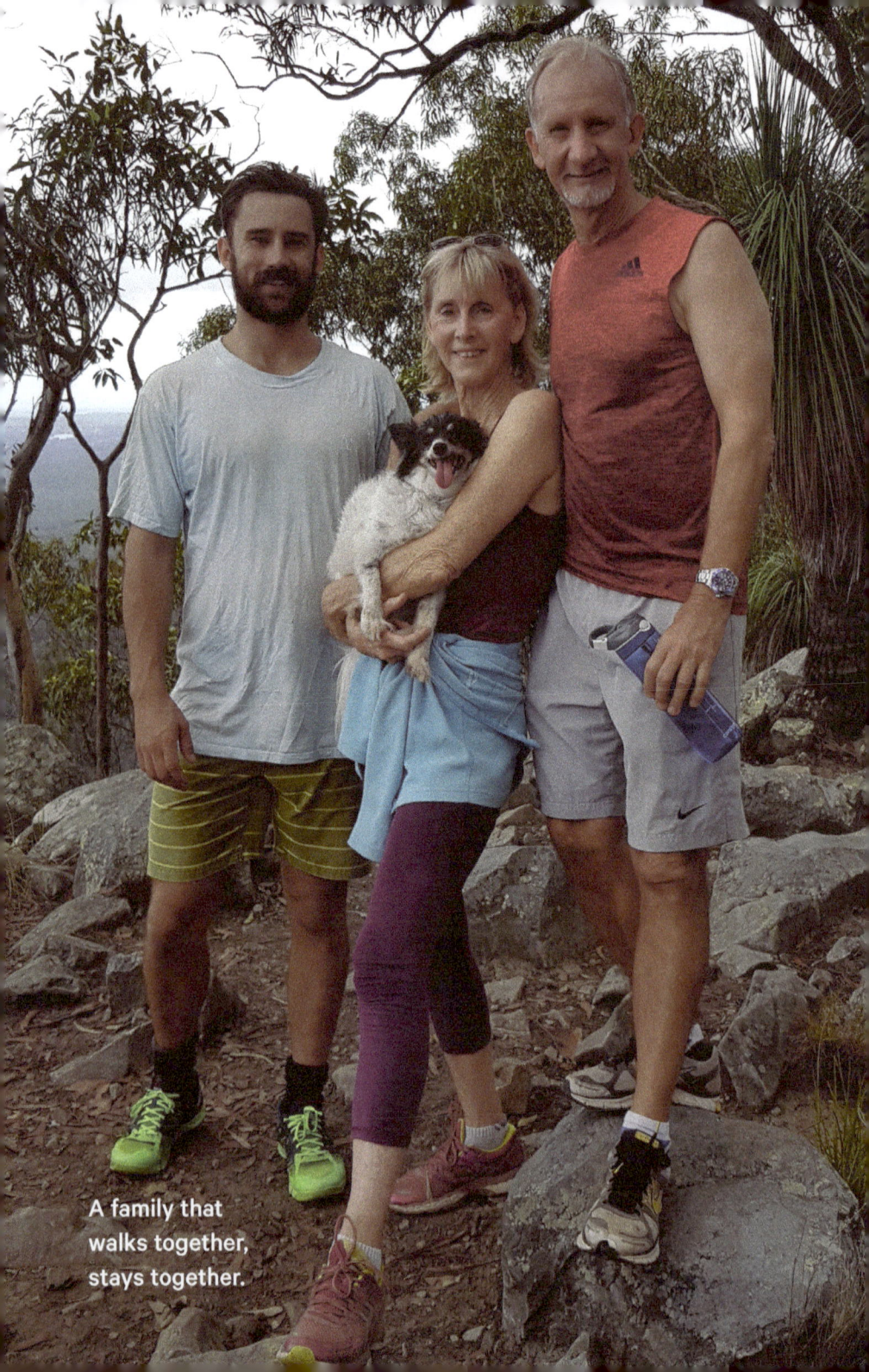
A family that walks together, stays together.

 # Walking

Instead of writing about different types of exercise, I decided to focus on the perfect exercise which is walking.

Most people still believe that for exercise to be really beneficial and improve cardiovascular fitness it has to be strenuous, so that you are drenched in sweat with your heartbeat well over 100 beats per minute. I'm here to tell you that you don't have to strain, and I'm pleased to say that research can back me up.

Brisk walking, not huffing and puffing, not marathon racing, has the same benefits of running without the all-too-common body bash that can come with it including knee injuries, hamstring tenderness and a sore back. I love running, but too much of it (like anything) can do me harm. Brisk walking uses more muscles than running. It avoids the jarring of running on concrete, which even the best running shoes only partially soften.

Striding along with deep, rhythmic breathing and arms swinging develops a strong cardiovascular system, improved muscle tone in legs, arms and upper body, and stimulates endorphin activity that helps the immune system. Walking improves lymph circulation, expands the energy field around the body and can be done outdoors on nearly any terrain or indoors on a treadmill watching your favourite movie.

Regular walking burns away excess weight, lowers blood pressure, improves the cholesterol profile, improves blood sugar and insulin dynamics, helps prevent bone-thinning osteoporosis, helps alleviate chronic lower back pain, improves mood and mental performance, makes you happier, relieves stress and improves posture. It can also help you come up with great ideas and solve problems, as it does for me.

Walking is natural and we are designed anatomically to walk. Sure, we can swim like a fish, we can run like a race horse, we can even swing like a monkey but the best movement of all is the walking movement.

I remember when I was child and walked 4kms to school in the morning and back home again in the early afternoon. I had to walk fast to keep up with my brothers who always beat me home. I learnt to be competitive then and I also became aware of walking and its effect on me, especially when I was fatigued after a full day of school. The prospect of the long walk home was daunting, especially to a little kid, but once I was underway it was wonderful and I made up names for the various houses and vacant blocks that I walked past. There was one house I watched slowly being built over a period of a year with bright red bricks and I distinctly remember the fear as I ran through my very own haunted forest. Years later, I checked out my old neighbourhood and noticed my haunted forest was now a three-bedroom brick veneer house with that instant lawn on the front – kind of sad, but I mention these stories to show how walking contributed to my life back then, just as it does to my life today.

Walking helps me to discover my own potential. It helps me to clear my head, remember things I'd forgotten while sitting down too long or being enclosed. My day is not complete without a walk. Now, don't nod your head and think to yourself, "I haven't got time to walk!"

You must make time to walk. It's even more important than feeding yourself, which I'm sure you don't have trouble with, do you?

People who remain physically active can gain many extra years of quality life and mental alertness to go with it. Sometimes I like to listen to music or a motivational podcast while I walk, but most times I just enjoy the peace so I can let my mind go on with its idle mind chatter.

For those of you who want to lose weight, one hour of brisk walking will increase your resting metabolic rate for a significant period after you have finished the exercise, continuing to burn off fat at an accelerated rate.

Finally, I believe that a vigorous walk will do more good for an unhappy but otherwise healthy adult than all the medicine and psychology in the world. Start walking today and begin a new life.

Great quotes to think about while you are out walking...

"Be kind, for every one you meet is fighting a hard battle."
~Plato

"If we don't take good care of our body,
then where will we live?"

~Anonymous

"If each of us sweeps in front of our own
steps, the whole world will be clean."
~Goethe

Anne Clark

"True change and higher human adaptation are not made by resistance to old habits. Change is not a matter of not doing something; it is a matter of doing something else."
~Da Arabhasa.

"If you have a weakness, make it work for you as a strength – and if you have a strength, don't abuse it into a weakness."
~Dore Schary

"We learn wisdom from failure much more than from success. We often discover what will do by finding out what will not do, and probably he who never made a mistake never made a discovery."
~Samuel Smiles

"Sense shines with a double lustre when it is set in humility. An able and yet humble man is a jewel worth a kingdom."
~William Penn

"What a man knows should find its expression in what he does; the value of superior knowledge is chiefly in that it leads to a performing manhood."
~Christian Bovee

"One only reads well when one reads with some quite personal goal in mind."
~Paul Valery

"If you give a dog a bone, he will take it. If you don't, he will go and dig one up!"
~Anne Clark

In the Raw

"I cried because I had no shoes until I
met a man who had no feet."
~Persian saying

"Probably nothing in the world arouses more false
hopes than the first four hours of a diet."
~Dan Bennett

"Pain is the most heeded of doctors; to goodness and
wisdom we only make promises; we obey pain."
~Marcel Proust

"It's better to prepare for an opportunity that
may never come than to have an opportunity
but find ourselves unprepared."
~Les Brown

"We are what we eat, think and say."
~Anne Clark

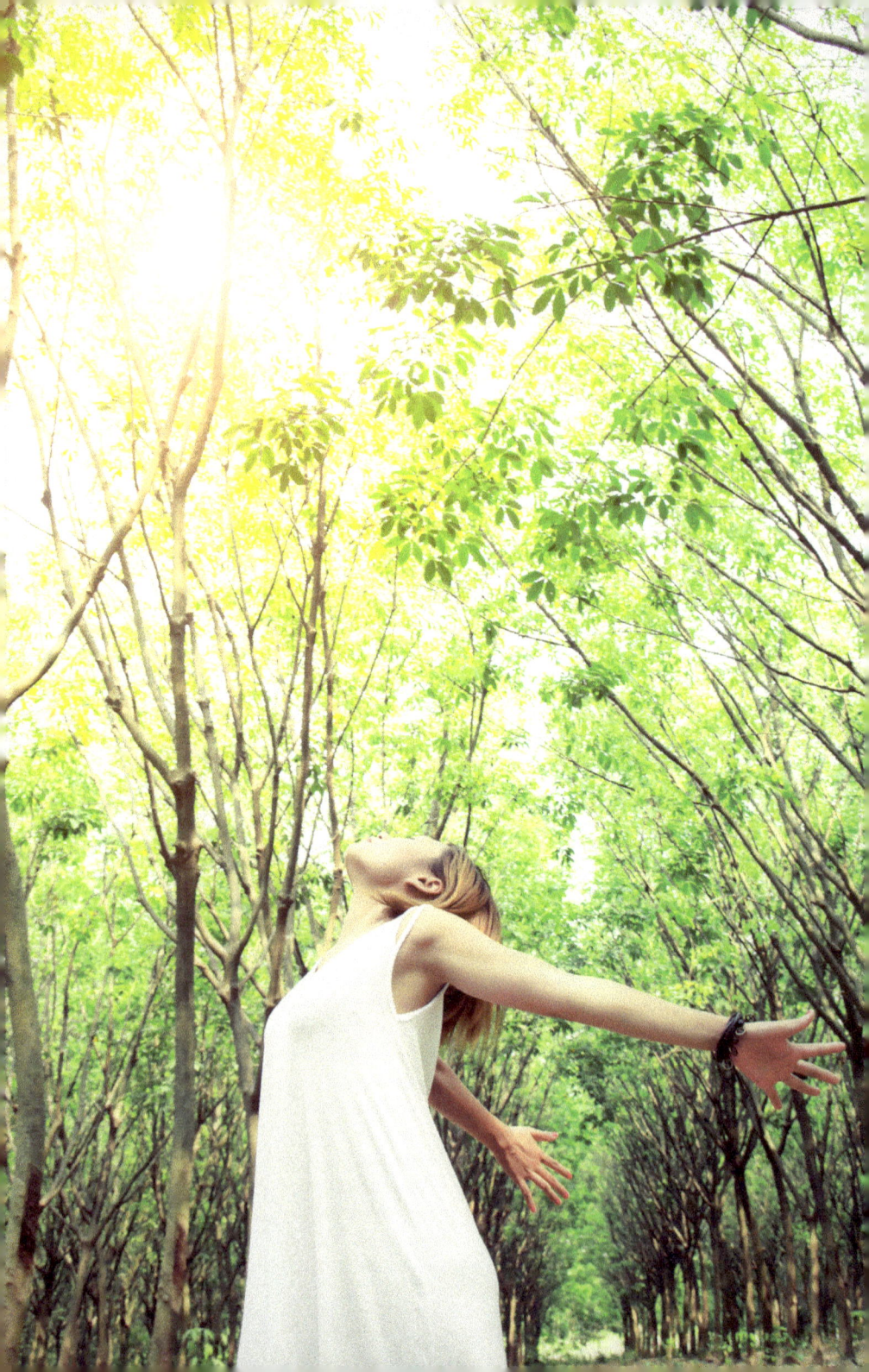

 # Breathing

I could write a whole book about breathing. Because it appears to be a purely mechanical process – we take in oxygen, nitrogen and other trace gases and breathe out carbon dioxide – we take it for granted. But breathing can also involve the conscious recognition that we take in energy, spirit and life.

A child's breathing remains open, relaxed, natural. As we grow older and fall prey to the stresses of life, both acute and chronic, most of us tend toward constricted, shallow breathing in daily life.

As we develop the ability to breathe deeply, as if down to the soles of our feet, we utilise one of the keys to cardiovascular health and help to prepare ourselves for any emergency situation we may encounter. By expanding our lung capacity, we actually breathe easier.

Notice your breathing right now. Consciously take three deep breaths, feeling your inhalation expand your belly and lower back, then your chest. Make the breaths very slow and deep, but not to the point of strain. Remember to do this at random moments in your day.

As you inhale, feel your body filled with vitality. As you exhale, feel your shoulders, chest, belly and entire body relax and let go of tension.

CONSCIOUS BREATHING

We can carry out conscious breathing anywhere, any time – it doesn't depend upon physical exertion. When you are waiting in a queue at the bank, stuck in traffic, waiting for an appointment or just listening to music, whatever. It has the added bonus of calming the mind and the emotions. Focusing on slow, deep breathing may serve as one of the most conscious and constructive ways to pass the time and is a key element in clearing obstructions in the body.

EXPANDING VITAL LUNG CAPACITY

Breathing to a count increases your ability to breathe slower and deeper, expands your vital lung capacity, and turns any rhythmic activity into a meditation. It may also help you to live longer.

This exercise can be done while walking, cycling, bouncing on a small trampoline, riding a stationary bike or engaging in any other rhythmic activity (except sex). It can be done as a sitting meditation to the rhythm of a ticking clock. I use walking in the following example as it is one of the best and most natural ways to apply the exercise. Within one or two weeks, you will notice measurable results.

1. As you walk in place, inhale for a count of two steps, then exhale for a count of two ("inhale, two, exhale, two… ").

2. Once you get the idea of breathing in rhythm to your steps, begin a regular, increasing progression. Inhale for a count of three steps and then exhale for three steps. Inhale for a count of four steps and then exhale for four steps, and so on.

3. Continue in this manner, increasing the number of steps, until you reach your comfortable limit, then work your way back down.

If you got as high as inhaling and exhaling to a count of twelve steps, go back to eleven, then ten, and so on until you reach a very comfortable pace (say, four steps), then maintain that pace. For shorter walks, you can go up and back down by twos.

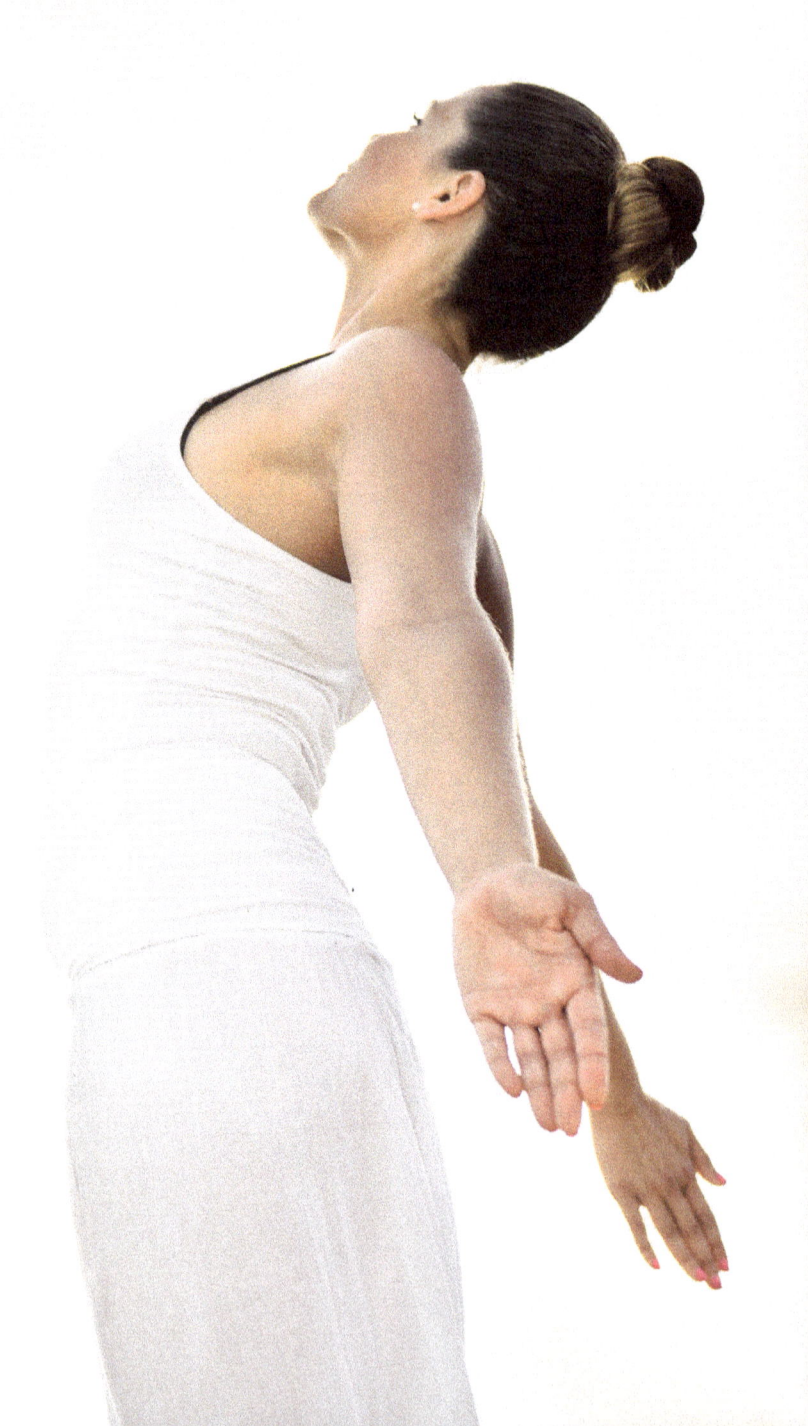

Posture and alignment

For many of us, 'proper posture' means sitting up straight. There is more to it than that. The phrase actually refers to our body's natural relationship with the force of gravity. Our body's skeletal structure is designed to balance vertically, like building blocks placed directly over each other. If we move one or two of those blocks out of alignment and push down from the top, the structure is liable to fall apart. This can happen more slowly to our body, over time, in the field of gravity.

Poor posture wastes energy and imposes undue strain on the muscles because they have to tense chronically to hold up parts of the body (such as the head) that are out of alignment. Misaligned posture contributes to many chronic headaches, neck aches, backaches and so on.

The following exercises and suggestions should help you to have a strong posture and maybe even better digestion.

- Sit hunched over and try to take a deep breath. Now sit up straight but relaxed and take a deep breath. Feel the difference.

- When you sit, stand and walk, imagine a string attached to the top rear of your head, pulling you skyward. Do this in a relaxed way and feel your entire spine lengthen.

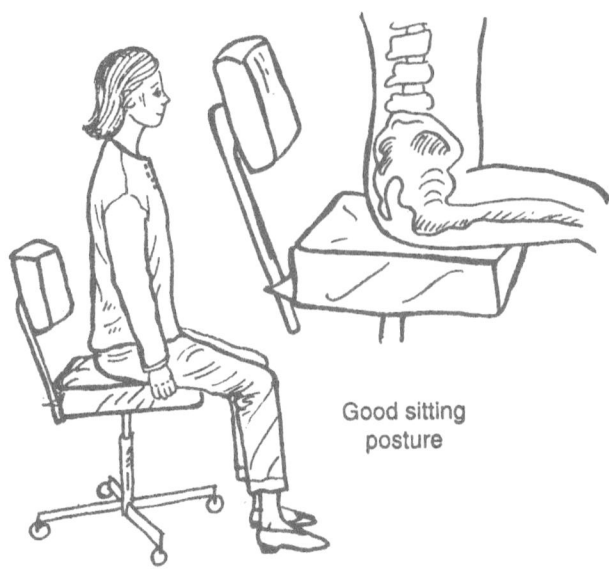

Good sitting posture

- When you sit or stand for more than a few minutes, shift your position regularly.

- When you sit and bend forward (at a desk, for example), bend forward from the hips with a straight back rather than hunching over.

- In general, notice your posture at least once each day. In a relaxed way, make friends with gravity.

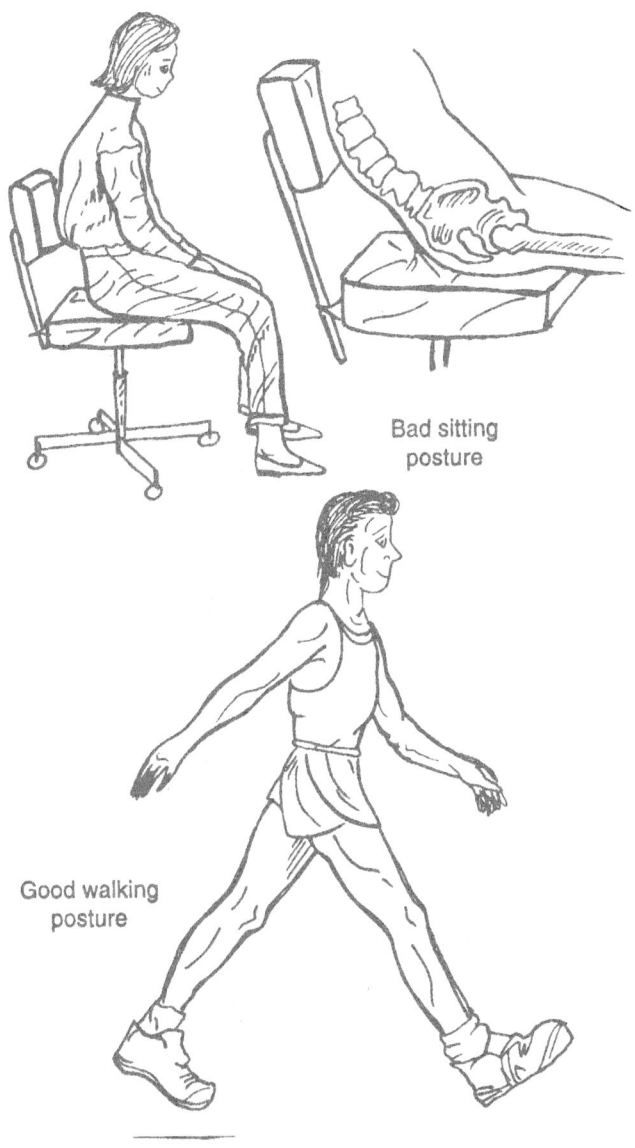

Bad sitting posture

Good walking posture

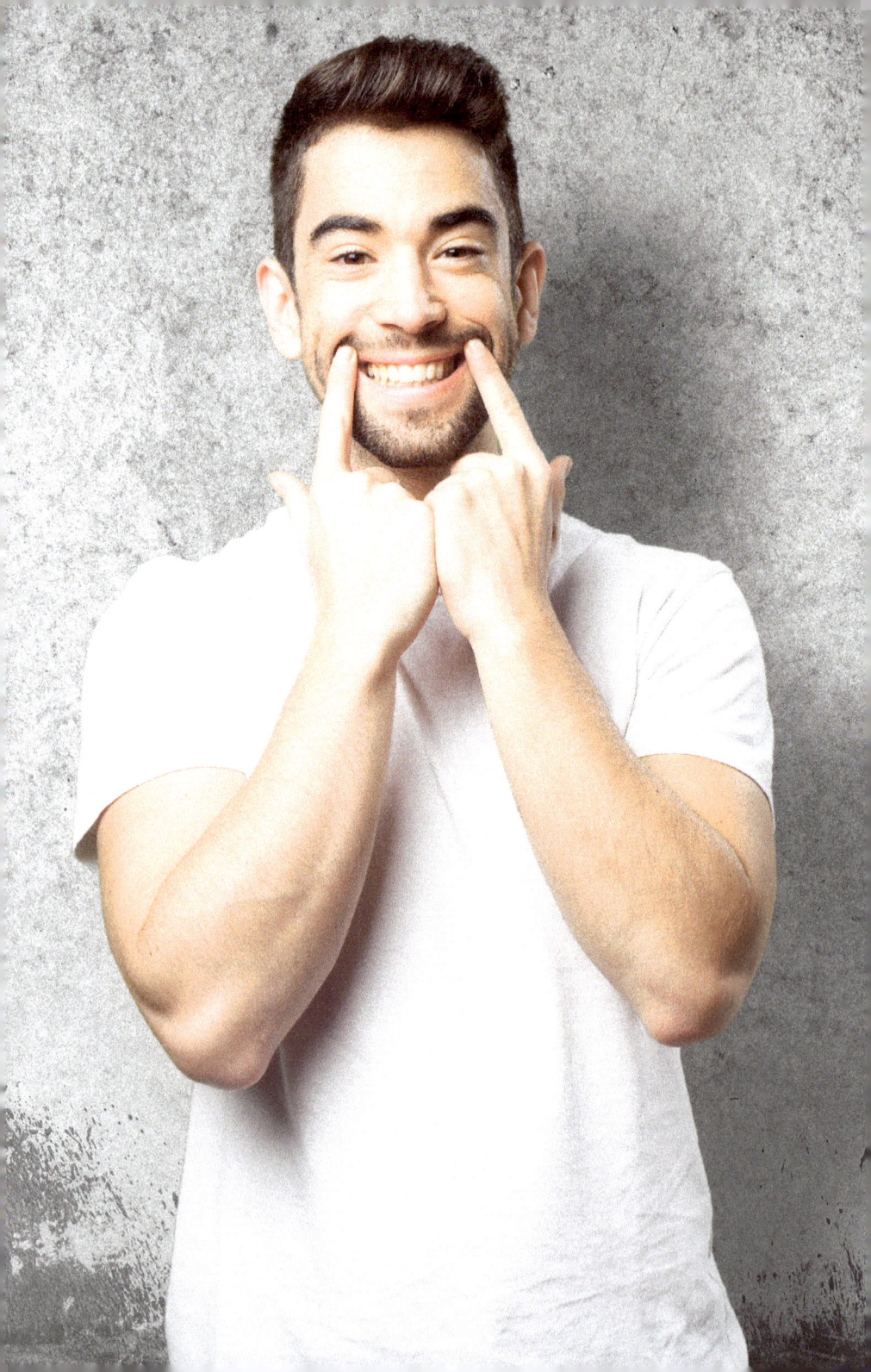

 # Teeth

In overall health, I feel it is important to mention dental care. Without our teeth we are very limited in what we can eat, and the appearance of your teeth can make or break your smile. Keep them clean and keep them strong.

Plaque reacts with sugar to form an acid which attacks tooth enamel and causes cavities. To make sure that plaque does not have time to build up or make acid, clean your teeth and gums at least twice a day. After breakfast and before going to bed are the best times.

It is important to brush at the correct angle and you don't necessarily need to use toothpaste. It is important to massage your gums whilst brushing your teeth. This can strengthen your gums and removes any food particles trapped underneath. Spend about ten seconds on each tooth before moving to the next one. Don't forget to brush the inner surfaces of your teeth and the biting surfaces of your teeth as well.

Normal brushing only cleans three out of five surfaces of your teeth. This means that the remaining two surfaces (between your teeth) need special attention. To clean effectively in these areas you need to use dental floss. Flossing is just as important as brushing your teeth. If you don't know how to floss the following brief description should be helpful but consult a dentist for professional dental care and advice.

How to floss: Break off 45cm of floss and wind it around the middle fingers of each hand. Guide the floss between the teeth. Never snap the floss between the teeth or into the gums. Use a gentle up and down motion along the side of each tooth to scrape away the plaque. Slowly move the floss away from the gum by scraping the side of the tooth. Repeat this process for all the teeth, including the back of the very last molar.

Teeth are meant to last a lifetime. Dentists have been bringing this message to their patients for years, but it's like a lot of things in that you only realise how important your teeth are when you don't have them!

A diet high in raw, unprocessed foods and regular visits to the dentist will ensure that you will still be munching with your own teeth well into the mature years. Your smile will be bright and you will always enjoy your food knowing that your teeth are strong and healthy.

Fasting... gain control of an out-of-control life!

If you read the Detoxification section in this book, you will already have an understanding about the powerful body cleansing process of fasting.

How often do you experience an unclear head, upset or bloated stomach, menstrual cramps, aches and pains, constipation or dizziness, and just carry on as though it were a normal part of life? Do you have offensive body odour, an uncontrolled temper, constant tiredness or feeling of worthlessness? Are you addicted to sweets, coffee, cigarettes and starches? Do you overeat or eat out of habit rather than because you are hungry? Do you have mucus in your throat, an acidic, bitter or salty taste in the mouth, encrustation on your eyes or wax in your ears? Do you wake up in the morning with a stuffy nose?

I'm here to tell you that these symptoms are not a natural part of life. It does not have to be this way. These symptoms can be attributable to a diet that probably includes one or all of the following: dairy products, meats, fish, eggs, even grains. The blood, lymph and cells become saturated with abnormal mucus and the body tries ever so hard to discharge it through the organs of elimination. Quite often this is how colds are formed, rather than from a virus and so-called germs your associates spread, as many would think. A cold is the body's way of telling you to stop what you are doing and give it a break. Animals know when to stop eating and hibernate, but humans are sadly ignorant of the body's warning signs. A cold acts as a safety valve for relieving the bloodstream and the lymphatic system of congestion which can otherwise lead to catarrhal infections, tuberculosis and tumours.

The aim of fasting is to rest the body so that the vital force which normally would be used for physical activity and for digestion and assimilation of food is freed for cleansing and healing. Fasting is one of the most effective natural methods of rebuilding the body's own dynamic healing powers and overcoming many major ailments.

What you miss in the pleasure of eating, you will gain in a feeling of youthfulness and joy of living. It will improve your health and help you to be less of a slave to food. It will sharpen your wits and increase your beauty. It will help you to gain control of yourself in an out-of-control world.

If you are planning a fast, you should consider your diet in general and prepare yourself for a smoother transition by eating only organically grown vegetables, fruits, seeds and sprouts, and drinking plenty of fresh water for several weeks. There is a very sound reason for this. The body stores toxins because it has limited capacity for excretion and neutralisation of poisons. During fasting much of the body fat is rapidly used up, suddenly liberating stored poisons. If inorganic foods have predominated in one's diet, a urine analysis will reveal a high level of DDT and other pesticides. A gradual cleansing releases the poisons slowly, never overtaxing the capacity of the eliminative organs.

Reactions during a fast or cleansing diet will vary with the individual, depending on how badly the body has been abused.

Possible reactions include: nausea, irritability, headache, fatigue, aching muscles, sleeplessness, rash and, in rare instances, vomiting and open sores.

Common reactions including: heavily coated tongue, bad breath, loss of weight, periodic irritability and a sense of weakness.

These are all signs that nature is performing art and helping to make you stronger in the long run.

Problem areas or congestion in your body will determine the type of eliminative crises you will experience during a fast. For example, a congested lymphatic system may be cleansed via boils and open sores. If the reactions become too severe, break the fast once the crisis is past and repeat it several weeks later. I myself have experienced the discomfort of a huge boil in the area of my lower back. It was very painful and took a little while to heal. I welcomed it later when I learnt more about fasting and cleansing and marvelled at the body's great capacity to cleanse when given the chance.

It takes perseverance, willpower and self-control to overcome habitual eating. Many signs of discomfort will appear on the first day when the body starts its cleansing. Headaches and muscular pains are the result of released toxins which irritate muscles, nerves and tissues.

Generally, painful reactions are of short duration of no more than a few hours. Lie down and wait for them to pass. Periods of great discomfort could be a sign that the concentration of toxins in the colon is higher than in the bloodstream and the poisons are being reabsorbed. During the first three days of the fast, an enema should be used every evening to cleanse toxins from the colon; afterward as frequently as needed. As the body becomes more and more purified through improved diet and fasting, the use of enemas while fasting will become unnecessary. Baths should be of short duration in lukewarm water.

I always look at fasting as a rescue remedy when I feel I'm losing control of my own eating habits. I use fasting as a time to rest and avoid infections and viruses. I love the triumphant feeling afterwards which words cannot explain. You will have to fast to know what I mean. Your body seems to become more in tune with the universe and you become more in tune with your body. I recommend fasting to everyone and encourage you to read as much as possible on the subject.

 # Sunbathing

Every day you should take a short sunbath in the morning if possible. Discard all clothing to improve elimination and absorption of oxygen and solar radiation through the skin. If sunbathing is new to you then you are about to discover a very wonderful relaxing beauty aid. Notice I use the word *sunbathing*, not *sunbaking*.

Traditionally sunbaking is just that – baking in the sun – and this is not good for your skin and ultimately you. Sunbathing, however, is a wonderful way of tapping into the sun's energies and utilising the power of solar energy to cleanse and heal the body. The best times to sunbathe are early mornings and late afternoons, when the sun loses its sting and the sun's rays are less harmful. While fasting, the cleansing process can be improved with the addition of a sunbath. Start by exposing one side of the body to the sun for 10–15 minutes, then turn over and expose the other side of the body for approximately the same amount of time. Common sense will tell you how long is long enough.

For those who work a nine to five sort of routine, aim to utilise the weekends as body maintenance times rather than body abuse times. It's all a way of thinking and knowing. It will come to each and every one of you when you are ready. The more you learn about your body, the more you will respect it and maintain it the way it should be maintained.

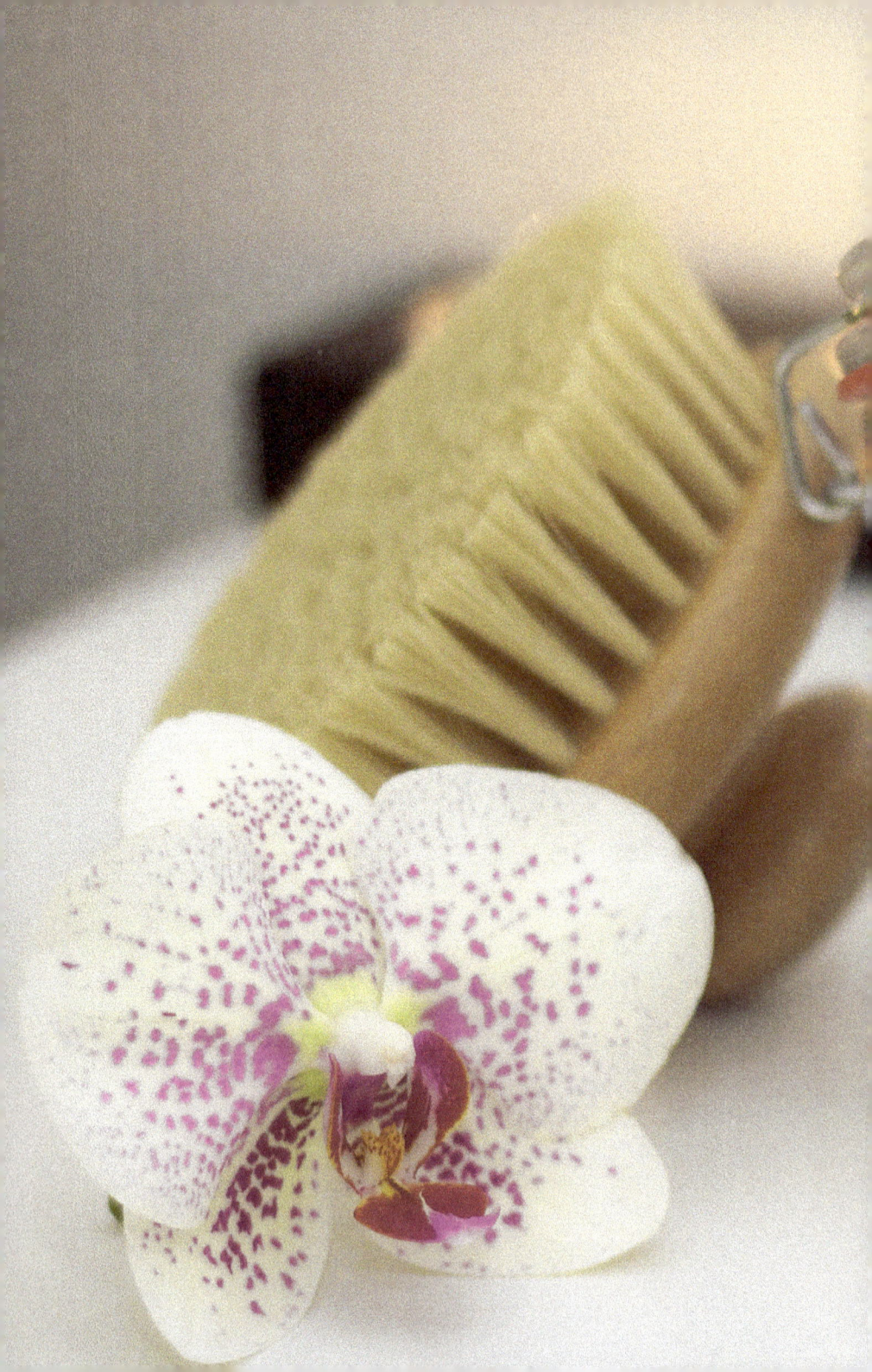

 # Skin brushing

Your skin is the largest organ of your body and is responsible for eliminating up to one kilogram of metabolic waste daily, healing and cooling the body, sensing pain, touch and temperature, and supporting and protecting the body.

To care for your skin, try a dry brush massage daily. This is done with a natural fibre bristle brush on a long handle which you can purchase from your local health food shop or pharmacy. Brush your skin vigorously all over avoiding the skin on your face and any rashes and damaged skin. Start with the soles of your feet, then brush up the legs, hands, arms, back, chest and, finally, the neck and scalp. Do it in this order for best results, and just before you shower. Dry skin brushing not only helps to eliminate toxins from your skin, but it also helps to stimulate the circulatory (blood) and lymphatic systems, stimulates the nerve endings and energises the body. This should take you five to ten minutes just before your daily bath/shower.

Every two weeks wash your brush with warm soapy water and dry it well. (This is the only time you will get your brush wet). For hygienic reasons do not share your brush with others. Why not give each member of the family their own brush for a Christmas present this year? A dry skin brush is a gift that will enhance beauty and give life and vitality. I believe that when you give a gift, it should be something that will help the other person, not take life from them. Think about the last gift you gave someone. Was it something of real value or was it destructive to their health?

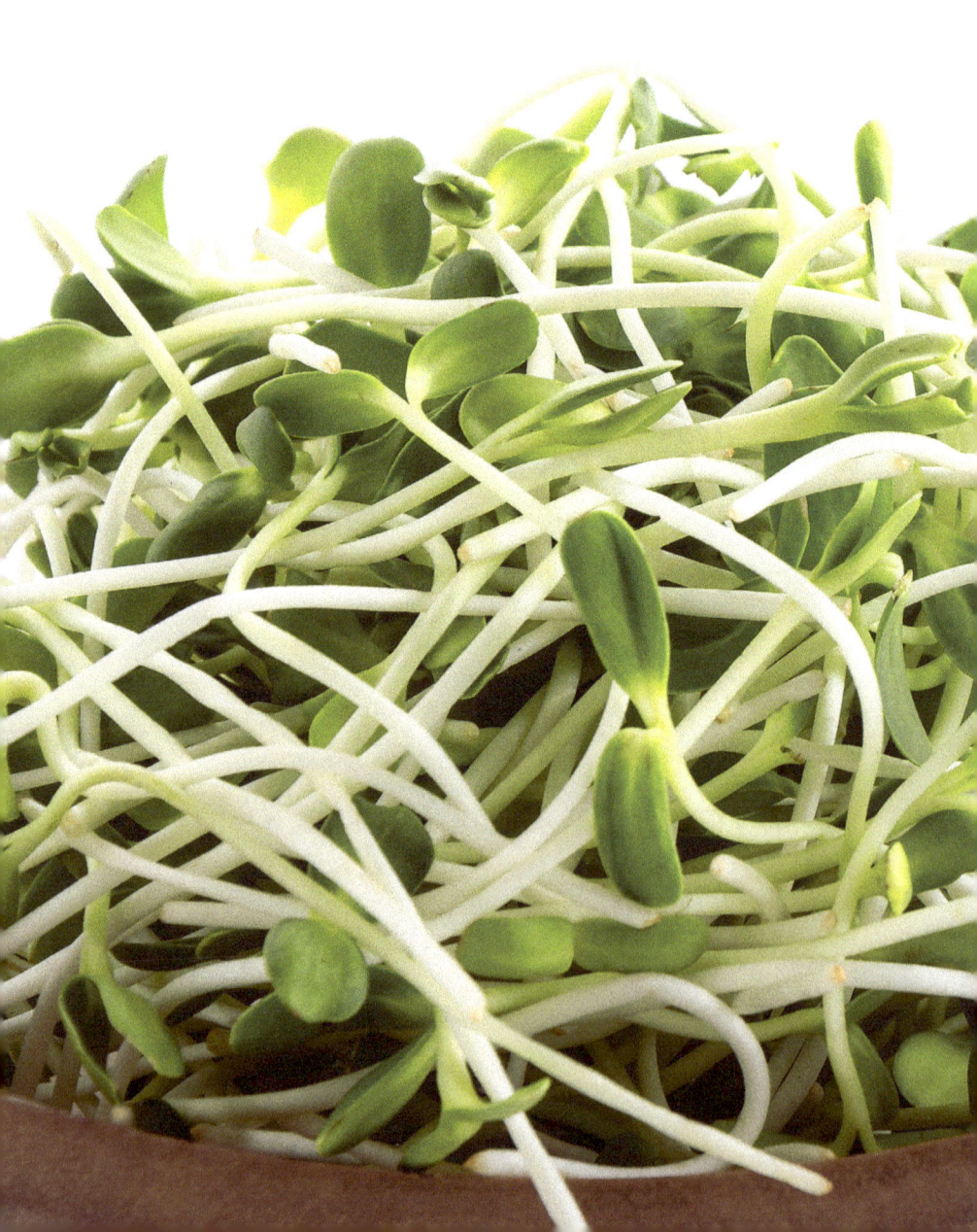

 # Sprouting

Sprouts provide the most nutritious and varied menu available. They are an excellent supplement to any diet and should be included in every meal if possible. Sprouts are extremely versatile and can be used as a snack, in salads and as a base for soups. In combination with other vegetables, sprouts can be juiced for a powerful energy boost.

Try to make your own it possible. Sprouts can be grown in any utensil without thought to soil conditions, climate, composting techniques and the worry of bugs. They are simple to harvest and easy to store for future use. They are not contaminated by insecticides or pesticides or made defective by heat, cold, preservatives, irradiation or ageing.

The soak water from most seeds is rich in water-soluble nutrients and enzymes which improve digestion. It can be blended with sauces and seed milk. Some of the soaked seeds can be used immediately. After three days of growth sprouts are ready for eating.

Considering the uncertainty of our times, it is good to know that you will be able to provide food for your family and friends and be assured good health. There is no survival food better than sprouts.

SEEDS FOR SPROUTING

For the highest nutritional value, buy organically grown seed. Make sure the seeds have not been treated with chemicals. If purchasing seed in small quantities, buy them from health food stores.

For sprouting, I use flat trays, but avoid trays made from soluble toxic metals such as aluminium, copper and iron.

Grains such as wheat, rice, barley, oat, and rye should be sprouted for more than three days. By then they will have swelled to twice their original size. Aduki when sprouted for three to five days taste like fresh garden peas. Mung, soy, lentil, peas and radish are most palatable in three or four days when they are still sweet and tender. When grown for six or more days, and exposed to light the last three days, they are beautifully green, but become fibrous like a plant and somewhat tough unless cooked. Chickpeas are at their best in two days. Most nuts, if fresh and alive in their shells, can be brought to their former tree-ripened vintage by several days of sprouting. Sesame, flax and chia are best after 24 hours of germination. Sesame develops a bitter taste if sprouted much longer. Alfalfa, clover, and fenugreek are at their best after at least one week of sprouting. Sunflower and pumpkin sprouts are ready in two to four days and are tastier than the dry seed.

SPROUTING METHOD

1. Rinse seeds thoroughly then soak them in a container of tepid distilled or untreated water (at least two parts water to one part seed). Place a nylon or cheesecloth mesh on top of the jar and keep it in place with a rubber band. The smaller the seed, the shorter the soaking period. Alfalfa seed does well with three

hours soaking but will not be harmed by 15 hours soaking. Larger seeds (chickpea, mung, etc.) may be soaked up to twenty hours.

2. After the initial soaking, drain off the water. Wash the seed and pour off the water. Place the container in a dark warm spot to hasten growth.

3. Twice daily the seed should be rinsed with tepid water. Pour the water directly into the container, then let it drain off. If not using a jar with a screen, use a fine mesh strainer to aid in pouring off the water without losing any seed. Seed hulls float or sink and can easily be removed. They can cause the sprouts to spoil prematurely.

4. Sprouts can be stored in the refrigerator, where they will continue to grow very slowly. If you have to be away from home for several days and have started a batch of sprouts, then refrigerate them before you go and then on your return the sprouting process may be continued to completion, and you will have all the nutrients you will ever need!

5. So now your sprouts are ready to eat and enjoy. Remember sprouts have different storage times in the refrigerator. For example, you will notice that mung beans have a short lifespan once sprouted to maturity and alfalfa sprouts will keep for several days and often up to a week in the refrigerator.

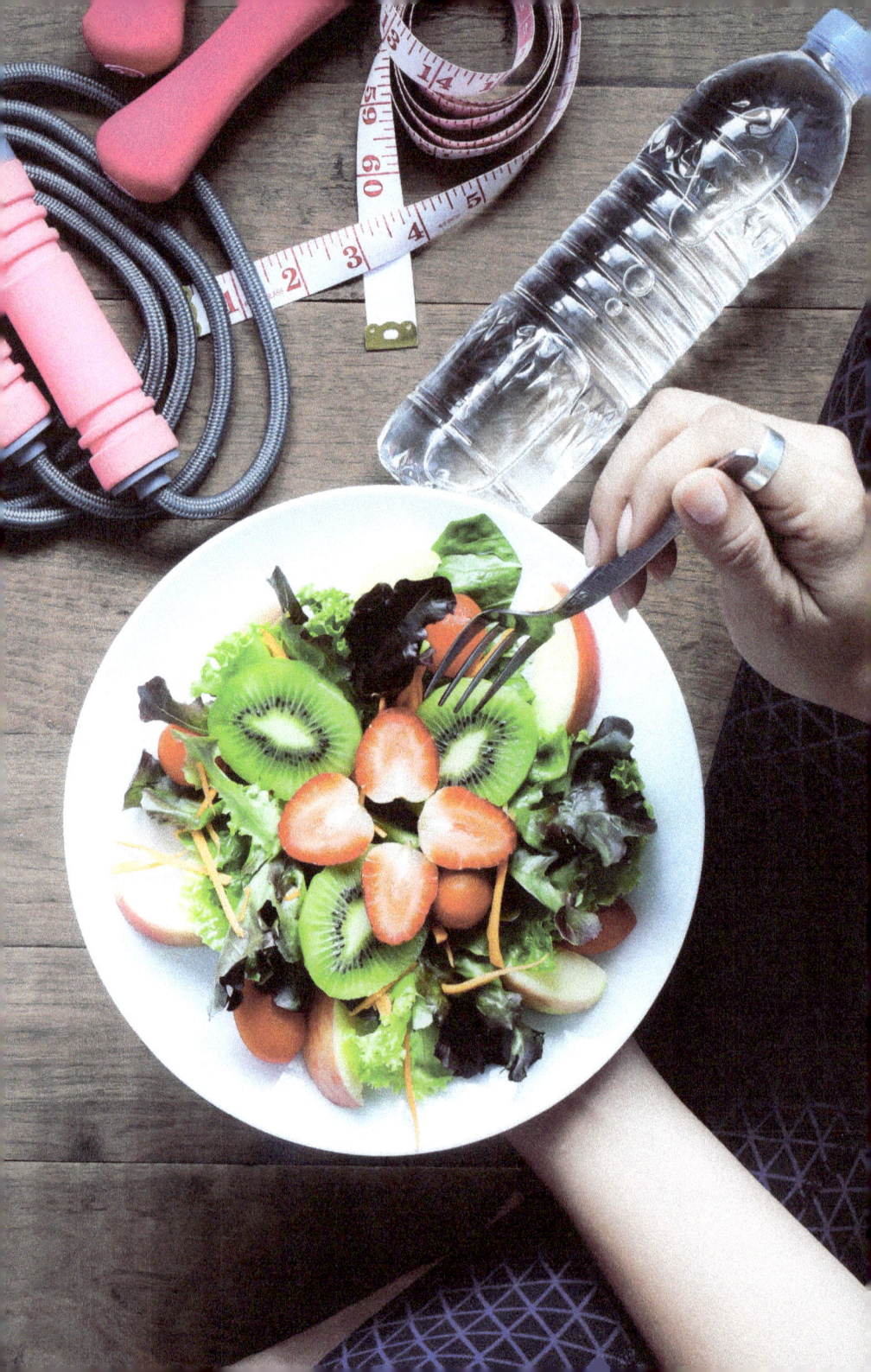

Living health – ten daily health acts

You have come a long way since the beginning of this book. You have probably detoxified or fasted, even if just for one day. You have experienced new taste sensations by following my recipes. You are more aware of the value of exercise and the benefit of living food and you will have discovered how wonderful it is to lie out in the sun without the constraints of clothing. You have adopted some breathing techniques that will contribute to a more relaxed, energetic you, and you should be hungry for more information and more enlightenment on the subject of self and health.

Now, how do we put it all together? How do we maintain 'Living Health'?

There are many distractions around us which make it hard to stay on the right path. Quite frankly, the only way to keep it all together is to try our best, become aware of our food sources and read everything we can get our hands on about health and nutrition. Those outside influences and distractions which take us from our quest for health can be eliminated simply with a change of mental state. Recognise the environment which causes you to stray off the track and put yourself back on course.

THE TEN DAILY HEALTH ACTS

These ten daily health acts are not meant to be rules; they are merely suggestions that will help you stay on the right track. They can fit neatly into your daily routine and enhance your life.

1. As soon as you get up in the morning, SMILE. That's right, smile to yourself in the mirror and say something good about yourself like: "You're looking good, honey!" or "You are capable of anything today!" or "My skin is clear and my eyes are bright. Today all things will turn out right!" I just made that up...pretty good, hey! Now your skin may not be clear and your eyes may not be bright, but it is amazing what happens when you use a little reverse psychology on yourself.

2. Before you retire at night, make sure there is adequate air flowing into your bedroom. Open the window enough so that fresh air can circulate. This will help you to detoxify while you sleep. If it is cold air, then simply place another blanket on your bed or snuggle up to your partner. You'll find a way.

3. Do some stretching before retiring and upon awakening in the morning. It is also useful to stretch during the day, particularly if you work behind a computer or desk for several hours. You really need to stand up and shake out your arms and legs. Take time to do this and you will notice that you can work with little discomfort.

4. Do regular deep breathing. See the Breathing section for more information.

5. Eat 75% of your food raw if possible and be sure to avoid tea, coffee and all dairy products.

6. Walk or do some form of exercise for at least 30 minutes each day. You know what they say: "Use it or lose it!!"

7. Take time out to be quiet, think, meditate. Preferably it should be the same time each day. I try to think quietly about nothing for at least five to ten minutes just before I go to sleep. This is good therapy and ensures a good sleep. Never go to sleep with bad feelings in your heart. Try to sort things out before they get out of hand.

8. Dry skin brush before you wash. See the Skin Brushing section for more information.

9. Drink plenty of water. Ideally drink water 15 minutes before a meal and 1 hour after a meal.

10. Do something nice for someone else.

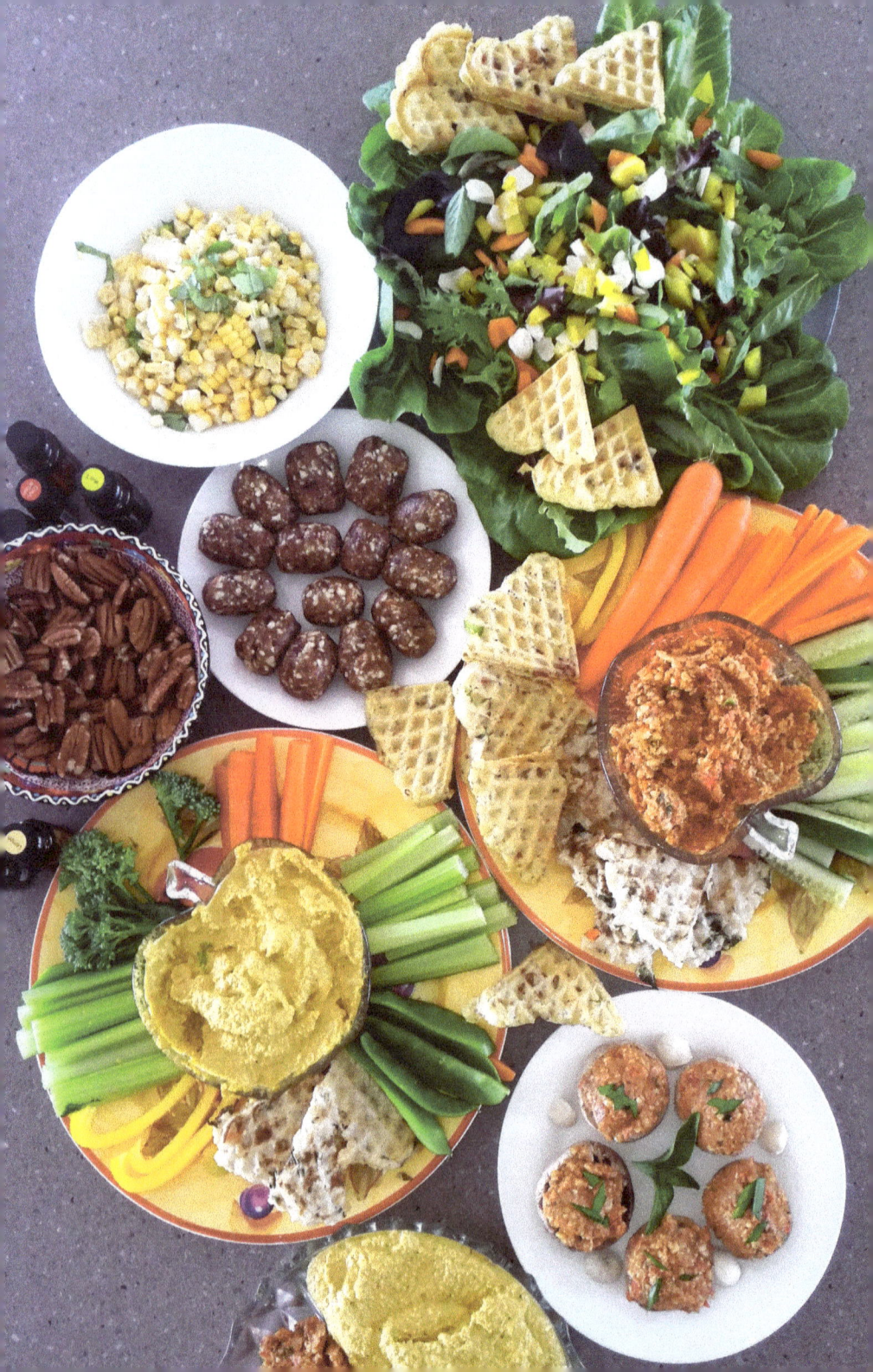

 # Recipe Index

ABC Mix   110
Alfalfa Fudge   178
Almond Cream   142
Almond Sultana Slice   203
Almond Sunflower Spread   197
Almond Vegetable Spread   136
Anne's Waldorf Salad   116
Annie's Classic Midday Muesli   112
Annie's Classic Peanut, Vegetable and Miso Spread   135
Annie's Dip Biscuits   147
Apple and Beetroot Juice   202
Apple and Orange Velvet   97
Apple Cordial   99
Apple Crumble Pie   180
Apple & Fig Slice   169
Apple Pear Juice   98
Apple Sauce   141
Apple Tahini Dressing   127
Apricot Coconut Bars   175
Apricot Fruit Spread   192
Autumn Salad   122
Avocado & Almond Supreme   154
Avocado Dressing   130
Avocado Spread   139
Avocado Surprise   100
Avocado Surprise Salad   124

Banana Carob Cream   186
Banana-Date Pie   165
Banana Mango Whip   85

Banana Passionfruit Ice Cream Whip   91
Banana Truffles   165
Beetroot Side Salad   116
Blueberry Whip   109
Brain Smoothie   100
Bumpy Carob Slice   195

Cacao, Chia Seed & Coconut Cream Mousse   189
Cacao Fruit & Nut Balls   190
Carob Apple Cake   191
Carob Bread   145
Carob Date Balls   208
Carob Fudge   170
Carrot and Celery Cocktail   98
Carrot And Honey Dressing   131
Cashew Mayonnaise   128
Cashew Spread   134
Celebration Bread   150
Celebration Cake   179
Celery Nut Loaf   157
Citrus Salad   109
Clifton Dressing   129
Coconut Cream   190
Crackle Pop!   185
Creamy Nut Dressing   130

Date and Apricot Jam Spread   140
Date Pecan Rolls   192
Date Shake   103

Dates with Orange   167
Delicious Mango Pie   182

Energy Lift Smoothie   102

Falafel Flat Bread   146
Fatique Rescue   104
Flat Crackers   148
Flax Seed Pudding   205
Fruit Bites   176
Fruit & Carob Fudge   170
Fruit Cup   87
Fruit Kababs   176
Fruit & Nut Bar   175
Fruit Pie Crust No.1   163
Fruit Pie Crust No.2   164
Fruit Salad   108
Fruit & Seed Bar   171

Gazpacho Soup   196
Grain Drink   201
Green Salad   125

Happy Drink   95
Hazelnut Loaf   155
Hazelnut Rough   172
Hollywood Bananas   168
Honey-Cinnamon Spread   140
Honey-Peanut Dressing   132

Ice Cream   186

Lazy Salad   195
Lemon-Limeade Smoothie   103
Lemon Oil Dressing   131
Luncheon Salad   125

Main Attraction Salad   166
Mango Passion Smoothie   95
Melon Salad   109

Nut Loaf   160
Nut Milk Shake   106
Nutty Pumpkin And Snow
    Pea Salad   119

Oat Waffles   200
Oriental Dressing   129
Overnight Fruit Tart   181

Paradise Whip   90
Patties   156
Pawpaw Sultana Slice   204
Pawpaw with Snow   107
Peach Nibbles   193
Peach Whip   86
Peanut Halva   173
Pea Patties   160
Pecan Cacao Pie   174
Pineapple Crush   98
Prune Bars   194
Prune Whip   88
Pudding or Cake!   184

Quick Start Shake   94

Radish Spread   135
Raisin Truffles   183
Raw Carob Brownies   177
Raw Cashew Cream Slice   206
Raw Cashew Lemon/Lime Pie   188
Rock 'n' roll   93
Rootie-Tootie Salad   121

Runner's Lift Shake   106

Savoury Balls   159
Savoury Rice Waffles   198
Sesame-Soya Dressing   132
Sesame-Sunflower Spread   137
Sesame Tofu Crackers   151
Silky Sauce   141
Simple Breakfast Cereal   111
Soaked Muesli   110
Spark Up Drink   201
Special Garden Salad   120
Special Ice Cream   187
Spinach & Mushroom Salad   115
Sprouted Mung Bean Bread   144
Sprouted Mung Bean Salad   117
Sprouted Tabouli Salad   117
Squash with Basil and
    Sesame   158
Sunflower Whip   87
Sweet and Sour Marinade   132

The Blotin Smoothie   101
The Grape Whammy   92
The Mouth Spark   95
The Sprout Roll   153
The Zinc Dip   134
Tofu Cream   191
Tofu Miso Dip   133
Tomato Herb Dressing   131
Tomato, Mushroom and
    Basil Salad   118
Traditional Mayonnaise   128
Tropical Fruit Sauce   141
Tropical Madness   104

Unyeasted Bread   145

Vegetable Loaf   161
Vegetable Nut Loaf   157
Vegetable Platter   123
Vegetable Sandwich Spread   137
Vegetarian Pate   138

Walnut Dressing   127
Watercress Salad   118
What's in a Cup Berry Juice   105
Wheat And Rye Biscuits   149
Wholemeal Waffles   199

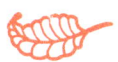

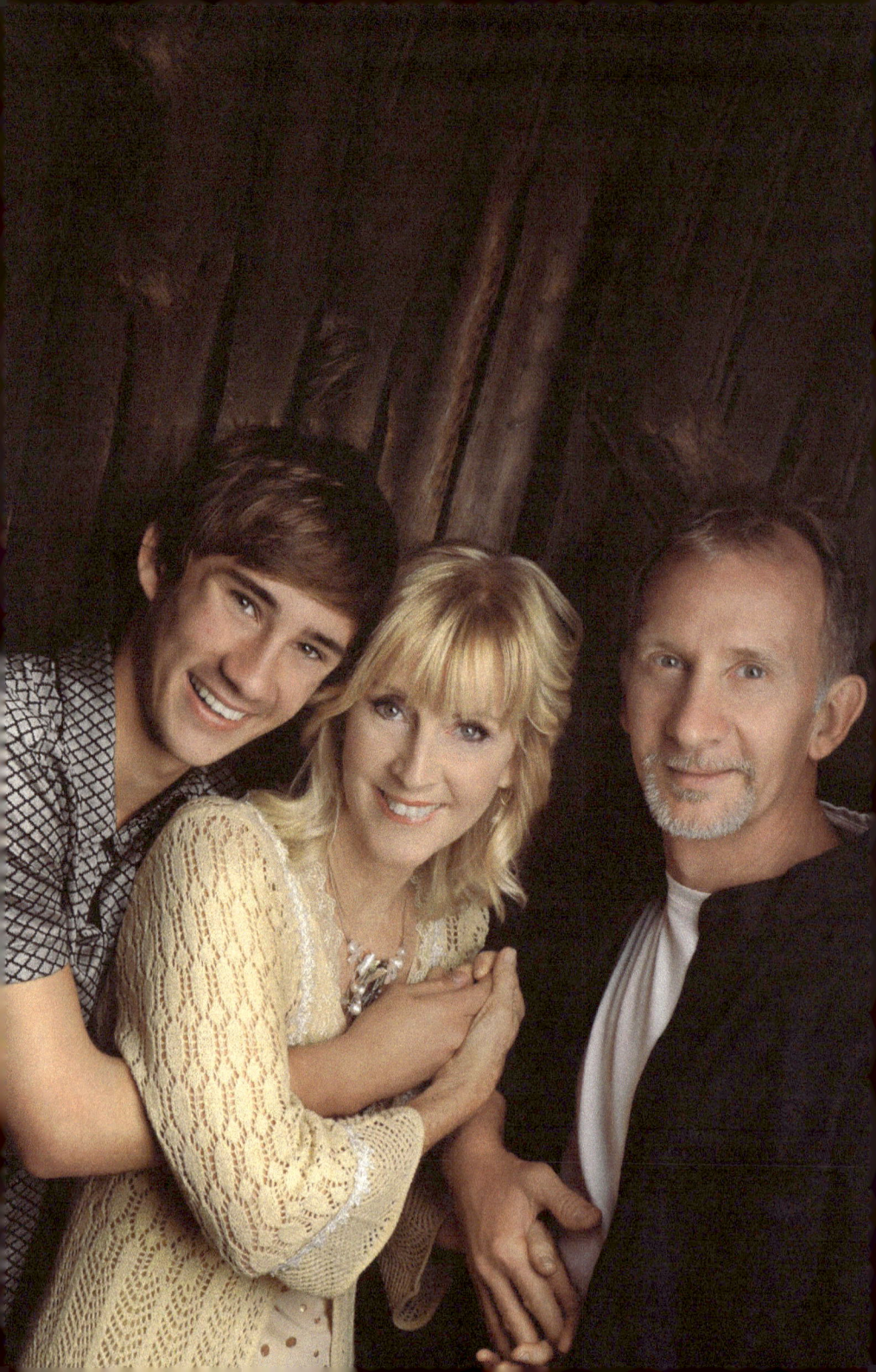

 # Other books by Anne Clark

All books may be purchased via www.anneclark.com.au.

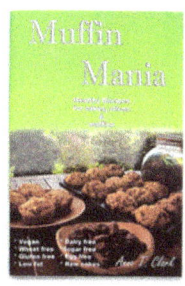

Muffin Mania

Delicious and tempting muffins that delight your senses. Simple recipes and lots of great hints!

Unlike the traditional muffin which is full of fat and dairy products, most recipes in this book are free from dairy, wheat, sugar, eggs and gluten. They are low fat and also suitable for vegans with a selection of sweet, savoury and plain muffin recipes. There are also cake and slice recipes included plus great hints on food combining, menu planning and exercise.

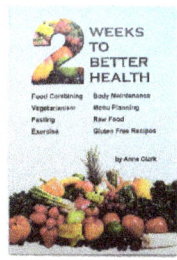

2 Weeks to Better Health

An inspirational and motivational guide on how to change some bad habits into positive strategies for life changing events and develop the confidence to explore better ways to live.

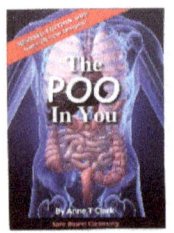

The Poo in You

Your bible for effective gut health to help you move into an arena of knowledge and safe practice – by cleaning up the rubbish...and putting it out for collection, so to speak!

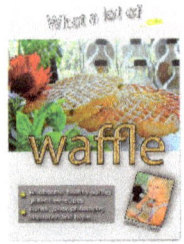

What a Lot of Waffle

Beautiful waffle bread recipes, which will be a welcome addition to any meal and any person. Recipes are gluten free and also free of harmful ingredients to the sensitive palate. Philosophy and stories that make up day-to-day existence in most households. This book will give you so much more than recipes.

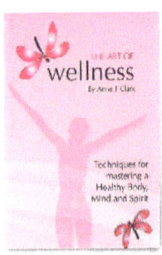

The Art of Wellness

The Art of Wellness is a compilation of contributions from over 15 health and wellness practitioners from the Sunshine Coast, Mt Isa, Bundaberg and Maleny.

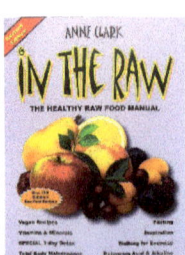

In the Raw (original edition)

In the Raw is about positive eating and intelligent food choices for healthy living.

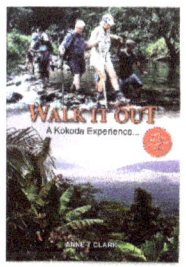

Walk It Out – A Kokoda Experience

For every walker, bush lover and history student, *Walk It Out – A Kokoda Experience* is a book filled with passion and respect for the wonderful land of Papua New Guinea and the people, the secrets that lurk behind every rainforest tree. This book is full of Kokoda Track history.

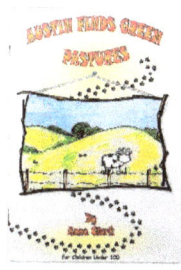

Austin Finds Green Pastures

Austin Finds Green Pastures is a children's book that explains how it truly is for the Australian dairy cow, the environment and consumption of dairy products.

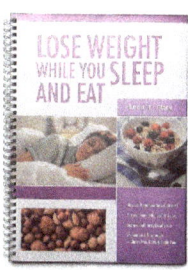

Lose Weight While You Sleep and Eat

Train your body to be more effective with metabolising body fat by getting more sleep, understanding the effects of hormones and how the different cycles of sleep are crucial to repair and maintenance.

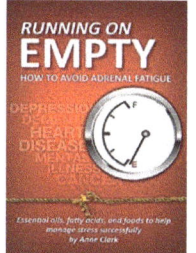

Running on Empty

Discover how to recognise when you are running on stress or pure adrenaline and why your body needs time out to calm your mind and support your physical repair and regenerate ability.

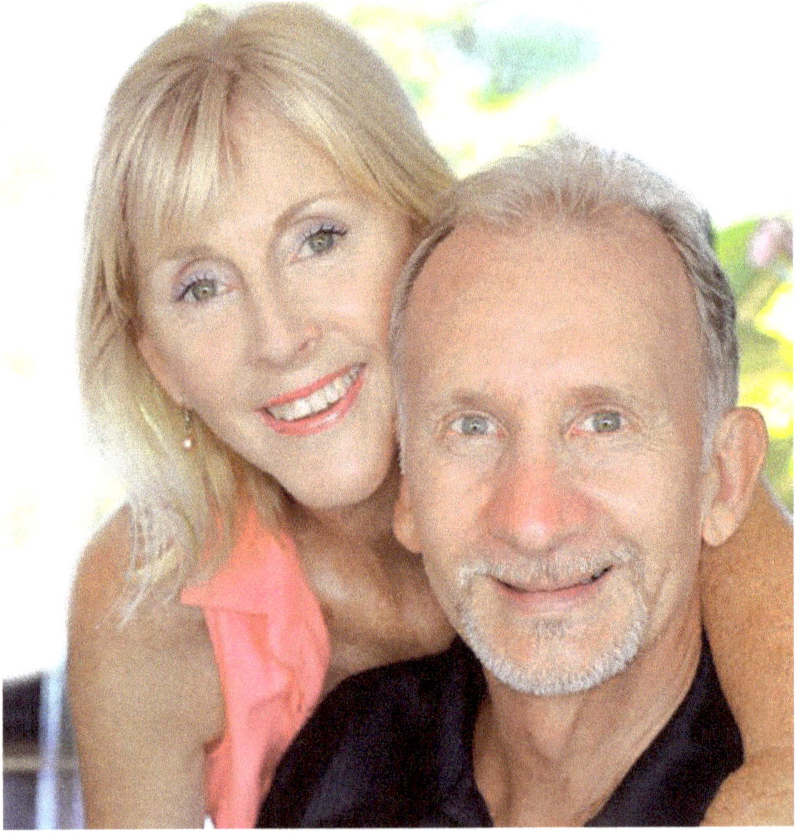

www.ingramcontent.com/pod-product-compliance
Lightning Source LLC
Chambersburg PA
CBHW040320300426
44112CB00020B/2823